Delivering Effective Adventure Therapy

Delivering Effective Adventure Therapy: A Therapist's Guide to Producing Transformative Change for Clients provides effective interventions for enriching therapeutic techniques using experiential methodology infused with metaphor.

Therapists continuously search for effective therapeutic interventions to engage clients in treatment and promote positive change. Adventure therapy overcomes the barriers of traditional therapeutic interventions such as, passivity, lack of input, and increased levels of resistance from clients. Rather than just "talking the talk" of therapy, this book provides examples and case studies that utilize experiences to enrich the therapeutic process and assist clients in reaching their therapeutic objectives faster with longer-lasting results. In addition to the practical therapeutic interventions detailed in the text, the theoretical background, rationale, models, case studies, and contraindications for these interventions are also explored. This toolkit is a practical and immersive guide which details adventure therapy practices in the field of mental health.

This text is essential for mental health clinicians, including psychologists, social workers, and family/marriage therapists, as well as therapists working in adventure, wilderness, outdoor, and alternative treatment settings.

Dr. Michael A. Gass, PhD, LMFT, CCAT, CBCC is the current Director for Research and Funding for Play for Peace <playforpeace.org>.

"Dr. Michael Gass has once again hit the ball out of the park in his most recent book on Adventure Therapy. This book demonstrates through metaphors, research, and a deep awareness of the healing process for adolescents. The reader will learn the power of Adventure Therapy through his unique writing style and his creativity for methodology, philosophy, and therapeutic interventions. Dr. Gass is a leader in the field, and we hope he will take us on another journey."

Craig Dobkin, *co-founder, Play for Peace*

"Dr. Michael Gass lives and breathes metaphor. His heart, passion, and depth for teaching are reflected in the eyes of his students. His wry smile is the tell of the transference of experience into tangible change. His art is creating a new perspective, reframing intervention, and allowing experience to educate. Mike Gass connects us to the beauty and mystery of life."

Kim Neal Wasserburger, *MSW, Karl Rohnke Creativity Award winner,*
Experiential Creations Consulting

"Dr Michael Gass is a soul like no one you will meet in your lifetime. He is a true mentor. To know him is to have the privilege of receiving as well as observing his unwavering capacity for kindness, generosity, and optimism. He is also determined, focused, and a genuine visionary about how best to help others grow and find their healing path. Over 40 years of experience, research, teaching, and parenting have culminated in this richly developed book brimming with useful knowledge and vivid metaphors. Dr. Gass has positively impacted countless lives through his undaunted leadership and passion to serve others."

Elizabeth Carol Bounds, *co-founder / board president, Parker Bounds*
Johnson Foundation / Wilderness4Life

Delivering Effective Adventure Therapy

A Therapist's Guide to Producing
Transformative Change for Clients

Michael A. Gass

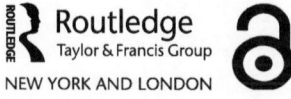

Routledge
Taylor & Francis Group

NEW YORK AND LONDON

Designed cover image: © Getty Images

First published 2025
by Routledge
605 Third Avenue, New York, NY 10158

and by Routledge
4 Park Square, Milton Park, Abingdon, Oxon OX14 4RN

Routledge is an imprint of the Taylor & Francis Group, an informa business

© 2025 Michael A. Gass

The right of Michael A. Gass to be identified as author of this work has been asserted in accordance with sections 77 and 78 of the Copyright, Designs and Patents Act 1988.

Trademark notice: Product or corporate names may be trademarks or registered trademarks, and are used only for identification and explanation without intent to infringe.

The Open Access version of this book, available at www.taylorfrancis. com, has been made available under a Creative Commons Attribution-Non Commercial-No Derivatives (CC-BY-NC-ND) 4.0 license.

Library of Congress Cataloging-in-Publication Data
A catalog record for this title has been requested

ISBN: 978-1-032-64028-0 (hbk)
ISBN: 978-1-032-64025-9 (pbk)
ISBN: 978-1-032-64030-3 (ebk)

DOI: 10.4324/9781032640303

Typeset in Times New Roman
by Taylor & Francis Books

This book is dedicated to the students, colleagues, and faculty I was fortunate enough to work with at the University of New Hampshire, Association for Experiential Education, Outdoor Behavioral Healthcare Council, and Play for Peace organizations. I continue to admire the learnings and perspectives they provide.

Contents

List of figures

About the author

Michael Gass (he, him, his) is the Executive Director for Research and Funding for the Play for Peace organization. Play for Peace is an organization dedicated to providing youth-led compassionate play to bring together people from different nationalities, religions, and backgrounds to find a common ground, build friendships, and create a more peaceful world.

Prior to this position he was a Professor in the College of Health and Human Services at the University of New Hampshire. He was the Co-Director of the dual degree graduate program (MSW/MS) at UNH with Dr. Anita Tucker. He is a licensed marriage and family therapist by the State of New Hampshire, recognized as a clinical fellow by the American Association of Marriage and Family Therapists (AAMFT), certified as a cognitive behavioral therapist (CCBT), and has achieved certified clinical adventure therapist status (CCAT) from the Association for Experiential Education (AEE). He received his Ph.D. from the University of Colorado at Boulder and completed postdoctoral studies in marriage and family therapy.

He is one of the creators of the Browne Center, a program development, service, and research center on adventure programming that serves over 10,000 clients a year with educational, therapeutic, and corporate clients. From 1988–1991, he created and directed Project Impact, an adventure therapy program for teens with severe emotional disturbances, and from 1992–1995, he developed and directed the Family Expedition program. This federally funded research project explored working with families of youth suffering from behavioral disturbances. He was the inaugural Chair of the Association for Experiential Education (AEE) Accreditation Council for its first 10 years and President of the Board of Directors of AEE in 1990.

Mike has made over 300 professional presentations and written over 200 professional publications in more than 20 countries. In 1999, the AEE commissioned him to write the adventure programming standards with Jed Williamson, which is currently in its 9th edition. He was also instrumental in contributing to the creation of the accreditation standards for the Outdoor Behavioral Healthcare Council (OBHC) in 2014, which is currently in its 3rd edition. His book *Effective Leadership in Adventure Programming (3rd edition)* (written with Dr. Simon Priest) has been the largest-selling textbook in the adventure programming field for the last 16 years. His book, *Adventure Therapy: Theory, Research, and Practice (2nd Edition, 2020)* (written with Dr. Lee Gillis and Dr. Keith Russell) is the largest-selling textbook in the adventure therapy field. His next book, *A Therapist's Guide to Adventure Therapy*, will be released on January 1, 2024, by Routledge/Taylor Francis Publishing.

Mike received the Association for Experiential Education's Outstanding Experiential Teacher of the Year Award in 1998, delivered the Marina Ewald and Kurt Hahn Address for AEE in 2002, and received AEE's Distinguished Researcher Award in 2011. He received the 2005 UNH School of Health and Human Service's Distinguished Career Research Award and the 2011 University Award for Excellence in International Engagement. In 2016, he was awarded the NATSAP Leadership Award, the OBH Eagle Award, and the TAPG Heart of Adventure Therapy Award. In 2018, he received the Harlan Gold Award from Cortland State University, and in 2023, he received the "Clan in the Hand" award. In 2023 NATSAP established the Michael Gass Research Award; this award honors Dr. Gass for his pioneering contributions in the field of behavioral health, particularly with adolescents suffering from issues of depression, anxiety, and substance use disorders. This is done by annually selecting the top research paper in the field of behavioral health.

Through all this, he has received unconditional love and support from his family: Cristina, Tony, Amaryth, and Andrew.

Preface

This book is designed to take you on a professional journey that could forever change how you work with clients in behavioral healthcare settings. And you should know whether to continue reading this book after reading the first couple of pages. Let's get started:

1 I am asking for no more than two minutes of your time. If you can't take two minutes, please place this reading aside for when you can take two minutes.
2 If you have anything in your hands (e.g., a cup of coffee), please set it down.
3 Okay, fold your arms, placing one on top of the other.
4 As you become settled with your arms folded, what words would you use to describe the thoughts, feelings, or attitudes you might be experiencing?
5 Next, fold your arms the other way, placing the top arm on the bottom and the bottom arm on top. Don't be surprised if getting into this new position takes some time. As you become somewhat settled in this new position, do you notice any different feelings, descriptions, or insights you may be experiencing?

You have just experienced a kinesthetic metaphor.

Kinesthetic metaphors are a vital component of delivering effective therapy, where...

- Intentional actions with isomorphic links to clients' affect, behavior, or cognitions aid in the transfer of learning through the clients' perception of their similarity;
- Therapeutic kinesthetic metaphors mirror clients' previous actions up to a point where the client's choice in the current action will lead to new learning and/or a break in dysfunctional behavior patterns; and
- Successful resolution of the kinesthetic experience provides insight/ pathways/clues to successful resolution of the client issue.

Are you interested in learning more about this enriching approach to comparing these different sensations, thoughts, and feelings?
  Read on!

Michael Gass
July 2024

Acknowledgement of Open Access Funding

The following Foundations have provided the funds necessary to cover the open access publication costs of this book so this information will be accessible to all individuals regardless of socio-economic status:

Parker Bounds Johnson Foundation
Routledge Press
Sky's the Limit Foundation
WoodNext Foundation

Acknowledgements

Without the support of Dr. Lee Gillis and Dr. Simon Priest, this work could not have been possible. I continue to walk and learn from these compassionate leaders. Thank you for your time, care, attention, and unconditional support. The fundamental text for chapters 3-5 of this book is the "Essential Elements of Facilitation." Dr. Priest, Dr. Gillis, and I are offering complimentary e-book access that can be obtained by contacting the Association for Experiential Education at the following address:

AEE
2315 18th South Street
St. Petersburg, FL 33712
303-440-8844

Introduction

I was asked to serve as a guest editor for a professional journal addressing current issues and practices of client facilitation. After sifting through, selecting, and commenting on the various pieces for the journal, I was faced with probably the most challenging task of all – writing an introduction that would embody the concepts covered in the journal as well as the current "state of the art" thinking on facilitating clients. Faced with this formidable task, I became anxious, worrying I might overlook some vital concept of this important process. I also became frustrated with my inadequacies and, as a result, was not the most enjoyable person to spend time with around my work or home. On one particularly grouchy, rainy Saturday morning, I was at home, mumbling to myself while staring blankly at my computer screen without any ideas on how to proceed. I was interrupted by my six-year-old daughter, who asked me to stop working and play with her. Fortunately, I was totally convinced my ability to produce anything of substance was hopeless and joined my daughter in her "agenda."

My daughter had encountered her own set of obstacles in reaching her goal. She had a soccer game scheduled for that morning, but those plans had been "washed out" by rain, and she was trying to devise an alternative way of creating a fun and productive Saturday morning. After surveying the resources around our house, she discovered 8–10 empty pizza boxes in our recycling bin as part of the residue from her brother's birthday party. She brought these boxes inside the house and arranged them (as well as our living room) into her understanding of what a "Pizza Store" would look like. After creating this environment, she decided that she needed someone to play with, and a "grouchy old dad" would have to do since no one else was around at the time.

As I entered her "Pizza Store," it looked like a messed-up living room with a bunch of pizza boxes on a bench. I had heard of pizza takeout places, pizza delivery companies, and restaurants where you could order pizza, but never a pizza "store." I asked her to explain the game. To my daughter, this was a Pizza Store where you needed to order pizzas over homemade cardboard phones, create pizzas with only the truly best ingredients (i.e., chocolate, cheese, and peanut M&M's), pay for the pizzas at the appropriate price (e.g., horseback rides on her father's back twice around the house), and always return the pizza carton after your order so the game could continue to be played.

When clients are seeking change, it seems to work best when therapists join with clients in a "story-like" editing process. The most important thing in helping clients edit their stories is to recognize the stories are the clients', not the facilitators'. In their stories, clients are both the actors and directors. And if these stories are meant to have any true and lasting value for clients, facilitators must recognize that the final version of the story (as well as the initial script) is the clients' and is one they will continue to possess after the facilitation experience is completed.

As I found myself at the Pizza Store again a couple of weeks later, I became more aware of my role in playing my daughter's game. I asked her if she liked or even minded me adding ideas to help her make a better story. She said that when I had some good ideas, she added them to her game. I asked her what she did with my ideas that weren't helpful as part of her story. She said she listened to them but didn't use them because they didn't "work."

This learning from my daughter reminds me of several critical features of utilizing metaphors as a facilitator. First, we must position and empower our clients so they can be in control of their own editorial processes. During our game, I highly valued my daughter's interpretation of our experience. I suspended my disbelief of the concepts foreign to me (e.g., Pizza "stores," chocolate and M&M's on a pizza) and looked to see how the integrity of such critical elements could be maintained in our experience. I also looked to my daughter as the "expert" in guiding our meaning and interpretation.

In the use of metaphors with learning experiences, some professionals (e.g., Mack, 1996) have criticized the work of others (e.g., Bacon, 1983) in their efforts to design metaphoric processes for clients, labeling such approaches as "imposing" facilitator metaphors and being inappropriate. Professionals like Mack are correct in their assumptions when such frameworks make little sense to a client's reality (e.g. when a metaphoric framework has little connection to a particular client's issues). In such times, the facilitator's story or set of "right answers" for clients takes dominance over what is the client's story or set of answers or outcomes. Mack's work reminds us that the editing process must include what clients bring to an experience.

However, it is equally important to remember that facilitating experiences involves more than just deriving a client's story. This editing process truly becomes a co-creation process involving both the client and the facilitator based on what these clients need. Such co-creation is usually necessary for functional change to occur (note that clients who would "self-facilitate" such change would generally not be seeking out the services of a "facilitator"). It is not an "either client or facilitator" driven process but a "both client and facilitator" editing process.

It was fascinating to be part of this experience because in this store, every time we came to part of the experience my daughter didn't feel was working out the way she wanted, she would change the rules of the experience, editing her story of what was supposed to happen. In her perception, we would "rewind" the story as one would rewind a videotape, editing what had occurred to create a better interaction and then continue the game.

Many facilitators (e.g., Freedman & Combs, 1996; Gillis & Hirsch, 1998; Nadler & Luckner, 1997; Walter & Peller, 1992; White & Epston, 1990) see the process of creating and facilitating metaphors in a similar way to how my daughter created and facilitated her story. People often embody their life experiences in this "story-like" fashion and strive to edit their life stories when they are not as satisfactory or productive as they could be.

A second critical feature that facilitators should consider when using metaphors is that the ideas we offer as facilitators might be helpful for clients, but they also need to be presented in an attractive or enticing way for clients. The primary value of the metaphor does not lie in some clever technique or structure but in the value and meaning to the client (e.g., Zeig, 1994). What also strengthens the metaphoric connection for clients is a recurring structure and insight in presentations, like a chorus from a favorite song one might find being played repeatedly on the radio.

Third, the unfortunate reality in some clients' lives is that they don't always find themselves in situations where their editorial processes are so easily self-facilitated as my daughter's Pizza Store, or in situations where what they "want" is not always what they "need." When this occurs, as facilitators, we must be even more attuned to what value system will make sense for clients in their present and future lives. We must seek to access and utilize client metaphors that can be re-edited and adapted once their lives begin to take on greater clarity. This seems vital for change to continue over the long term in clients' lives.

Full of knowledge from my daughter's Pizza Store, I returned to my computer later that day and wrote this narrative that has served as a storyline for me when using metaphors with clients. When I began structuring client metaphors in this interactive, co-creative manner, I witnessed the spontaneous development of change in my work with clients. I hope my daughter's story has provided insight into your own use of metaphors with your clients.

A version of this chapter was previously published in *The Journal of Experiential Education* (1997), *20(2)*, 66–67.

1   What is adventure therapy, and how does it work?

Behavioral healthcare professionals were filing into the conference room where I was about to lead a session on adventure therapy. I was both excited and a little bit nervous about how I would deliver my presentation in a way my colleagues would understand. As I glanced over the crowd, I noticed one participant who looked uncomfortable ("Maria"). Despite sitting in her chair, she was squirming and mumbling disparagingly about her conversation with a colleague ("Juan"). I asked Maria if something was wrong, and she shared that despite her efforts to explain the concepts of adventure therapy, she was having trouble explaining to him how this treatment approach could work with clients. And the more Maria tried to explain the topic, the more confused Juan became, which led to even greater frustration for both. I asked them if we could use some experiential methods to examine the situation and they agreed.

I asked them to sit in their chair, hold onto it, move it to the left and right, spin around in a circle, and go around each other. When I asked them what they were experiencing, they said they felt stuck, limited, and awkward in their chairs. Then I told them to stand up and perform the movements I had just asked them to do, but without the chair. They moved right, then left, and around in a circle, like before. I asked them how they felt and how this experience compared to their perceptions and understandings when they were "stuck" in their chairs. Juan said he felt freer and had more choices, while Maria spoke about how this could help a client make connections between the "chair activity" and their treatment plan.

Clients and therapists have found therapeutic success in many therapeutic programs by settling into comfortable chairs to talk about treatment issues for 50 minutes. These discussions evolve from the therapist's ability to access, dissect, and compile clients' insights, issues, history, etc., to co-create functional change and beliefs. Sometimes, this knowledge is invaluable for typical, in-office cognitive therapeutic approaches. But at other times, it can be limiting and build increasingly resistant interactions.

But what if you and your client got out of the chairs? Could treatment become increasingly richer, more effective, and better contextualized by the client?

DOI: 10.4324/9781032640303-1

Adventure therapy provides opportunities for clients to identify and learn from new perspectives. By getting their clients out of the chair and off the couch, therapists can open richer and broader possibilities for conducting therapy. As seen in Maria and Juan's story, an adventure experience (i.e., moving with and without a chair) was combined with a metaphor (e.g., What is keeping you stuck?) and guided reflection to begin insightful and functional change. Experiential therapies are not meant to replace traditional therapeutic models and structures but to increase potential outcomes for therapy by implementing kinesthetic approaches. Moving out of the chair can strengthen the client's insight and vision for functional change. The therapist can also gain richer experiences to reference with the client. When clients recognize and learn from novel experiences, they have more diverse perspectives to utilize when in session.

What is adventure therapy work, and how does it work?

Adventure therapy is "the prescriptive use of adventure experiences provided by mental health professionals, often conducted in natural settings, that kinesthetically engage clients on cognitive, affective, and behavioral levels" (Gass et al., 2020, p. 1). Adventure therapy experiences can be presented to clients of all ages, group sizes, and treatment needs. The key is facilitating the experience (i.e., initiative, activity) to meet client needs, capabilities, and other considerations. Elements of this psychotherapeutic approach can be found in the work of Milton Erickson (Haley, 1973), Stephen Bacon (1983), Virginia Satir (1972/ 1990), Gregory Bateson (2002), Hans Selye (1974), Viktor Frankl (1946), and Carl Whitaker (1978).

So, how does adventure therapy lead to positive change? Building off the work of Walsh and Golins (1976), Priest and Gass (2018), Russell, Gillis, and Heppner (2015), and Russell and Gillis (2017), here are five factors that represent the basic underpinnings of how adventure therapy creates therapeutic benefits for clients: (1) Experiential centered change, (2) Immersion into nature, (3) Enriched group process, (4) Challenging experiences, and (5) the Use of metaphor.

Experiential centered change

Adventure therapy turns didactic therapeutic analysis and interchange into more active and multidimensional experiences. It augments the verbal processes of talking therapies with concrete physical actions, multi-dimensional interpretations, and experiences. One common phrase that epitomizes this interaction is how adventure therapy clients "walk *and* talk rather than just talk their behaviors." When properly delivered, adventure therapy supports clients in achieving greater depth and enhanced therapeutic interaction.

Adventure therapy experiences are designed to direct clients to examine behaviors and their effects on their actions. When a therapist facilitates an adventure therapy experience, the opportunity to reflect and process the behaviors is ongoing throughout the activity. At the end of the activity, a formal debrief of the client's reflection and treatment understanding takes place.

Adventure therapy experiences may also reduce client resistance by placing clients in unique, appropriate, intriguing, and supportive situations. Practitioners use the concept of "contrast" to describe the growth patterns produced by adventure therapy experiences (Priest & Gass, 2018; Russell, Gillis, and Heppner, 2015, Russell & Gillis 2017). It is a respectful and prescribed process where clients are invited into unfamiliar yet simplified environments that are straightforward. "Contrast is used to see generalities, which tend to be overlooked by human beings in familiar environments or to gain a new perspective of the old, contrasting environment from where the client comes" (Walsh & Golins, 1976).

When using adventure therapy, the role of a therapist changes from being the central agent of change (i.e., the person who makes change happen) to being a facilitator of the change process (i.e., the person who "shepherds" the client in their change process). This shift allows the therapist to become more "mobile" to actively design and frame interventions for specific client outcomes, like the positioning of the Milan therapists such as Boscolo, Cecchin, Palazzoli, and Prata (Cecchin, 1987). In contrast to theoretical conversations that often occur in traditional therapy settings, adventure therapy involves actual experiences designed to be clear and recognizable and produce direct feedback for the client (Walsh & Golins, 1976). In this manner, the feedback provided by the therapist directly attaches to and informs the client's issues. A key principle that guides adventure therapists to use feedback appropriately is: "I am responsible **to** the client, not **for** the client." Clients who receive direct feedback and information gain greater understanding and personalization from the adventure experience.

Adventure experiences also provide rich avenues for forming connections to real-life experiences. Like the psychological theory of "projection," clients' unfamiliarity with adventure experiences can provide rich assessment information for the therapist (e.g., examining life-long behavior patterns, dysfunctional ways of coping with stress, intellectual processes, conflicts, needs, and emotional responsiveness). Such material can be valuable for planning treatment interventions.

When debriefing an adventure experience, clients receive immediate and specific feedback on how well they achieved the initiative's goals. For example, if a client has the task of drawing a picture from a partner's explanation, the clarity of the picture is partially related to one partner's listening skills and the other partner's communication skills. The therapist can utilize the feedback from working through a task to highlight targeted behaviors that address the therapeutic issues.

Immersion into nature

Research has shown that one unique strength of adventure therapy is the significance of the outdoor environment as a restorative agent for clients. One element is the formation of a state called "soft fascination." This occurs in nature when a person feels calm and has less mental fatigue because they are not involved in their daily obligations and routines (Kaplan & Kaplan, 1993). Awareness (e.g., mindfulness) emerges as individuals pay attention non-judgmentally, make sense of what they are feeling and thinking, and are more receptive to events and experiences with an attitude of openness (Kabat-Zinn, 2003). Nature also fosters an appreciation for the beauty and awe of the natural world. These elements foster the restoration capabilities of nature to serve as a functional model for change (Kaplan & Kaplan, 1993).

Multiple studies have found that maintaining inherent connections to nature is a yearning many people seek to experience (Roszak, 2001). The affiliation with animals and plants in a natural environment is called bio-philia (i.e., love of living systems). It has been found that when youth bond with nature, their health, self-esteem, social connection, self-relatedness, and joy are enhanced (Chalquist, 2009).

Getting away and simply being in nature promotes the enjoyment of the outdoors (Russell & Farnum, 2004). Similarly, clients in adventure therapy regularly state that being in nature facilitates reflection on the substance and direction of their lives. It has also been reported to be restorative and ener-gizing for clients who have anxiety and stress (Russell & Farnum, 2004).

Another element of nature that empowers adventure therapy approaches is the novelty or unfamiliarity of being in the outdoors. When clients begin any therapy, they often possess strong resistance to the change processes (Walsh & Golins, 1976), being labeled as "homeostatic" or "pre-contemplative." Adventure therapy practices often reduce such resistance because therapists place clients in supportive situations that are new and unfamiliar. One reason for this reduction is that clients do not know how to organize their resistance when in a "novel and unfamiliar state" (e.g., "the body does not know how to lie"). Social norms, alliances, biases, competencies, etc., are not typically dis-played when a client is initially in a new setting. Because of this, clients, therefore, tend to present their "true" selves rather than more "socially constructed" selves (Russell & Farnum, 2004).

Similar to how contrast was used to foster new discoveries with nature, contrast can also be applied to how the environment and adventure activities can challenge clients. These changes' unique, diverse, and ever-changing aspects provide invaluable resources for therapists (e.g., risk-taking, perceptive observation, asking for help). The discord created through challenging experiences presents unfamiliar experiences where clients must develop capabilities they typically were unaware of or did not use. When clients "try on" new behaviors, they encounter the first step toward integrating new behaviors into their lives (Priest & Gass, 2018).

The uniqueness of working through an adventure activity often results in spontaneous and creative responses. The spontaneity and creativity applied to solve an adventure initiative and the potential for successful outcomes help clients begin to recognize positive change. In unfamiliar or novel environments, clients are presented with opportunities to focus on their abilities rather than their inabilities. This solution-oriented perspective is common in traditional practices, and adventure therapy settings amplify the potential of its use. Adventure therapy activities carry a goal for completion, and therefore, clients are aware of what they are trying to accomplish or achieve (e.g., working together to figure out the safe passage through a maze). Even when the outcome may be incomplete, clients are able to state what they learned, practice new skills, and identify successes. This type of orientation can diminish initial defenses as clients complete progressively more complex tasks. Clients may tend to resist change when confronting problems, but through adventure therapy, they instead approach issues with an air of wanting to take on a problem-solving activity. Clients are challenged to stretch perceived limitations and discover untapped resources, strengths, and solutions.

Enriched group process

As mentioned earlier, adventure therapy activities can be presented to clients of all ages (therapeutic age) in group sizes ranging from one to 15 and for a myriad of treatment needs. For some activities, a specific number of clients are required, and environmental conditions must be considered (e. g., flat grassy ground). The activities can be completed inside or outdoors, with minimal or no equipment (e.g., twine, squishy balls) and time requirements ranging from 15–45 minutes.

Before a session, the therapist selects activities that will highlight and provide growth opportunities that focus on clients' specific treatment goals (e.g., collective consciousness, autonomy, trust). An adventure therapy session begins with an introduction of what will take place for the next 50 minutes (or whatever the time frame). The therapist then presents the therapeutic intent and directions for the activity. For example, "Today, you will be asked to work through an experience that invites you to accomplish something as a family without using words." Following the activity, the therapist facilitates a discussion (debriefing) of what occurred during the activity, the consequences of the activity, and the application of the learnings for the client's future. Debriefing can be used to focus on treatment goals and integrate new contextualized discoveries made by clients. Behavioral changes are motivated by therapeutic questioning techniques or identified as an "ah-ha" moment by a client in manners that connect the activity they just finished to experiences in their lives.

To foster an effective debriefing session, the activity selected needs to provide avenues for growth. For example, if a therapist wants to focus on trust between a cis married couple, the activity needs to frame and include elements related to trust (e.g., Do you follow through with what you say you will do?). Adventure therapy can occur with clients who come as an individual, couple, family, or small group. Group sessions can provide more diverse and numerous ideas when debriefing topics than individual sessions. In a group, clients pool their resources, share the benefits of this enriched environment, and collaborate on their strengths as a form of reciprocity. Adventure therapy also includes groups made up of different families. Groups formed with people from other households can provide valuable therapeutic experiences. Therapists must consider the treatment plans of each family and organize the activity and session accordingly (e.g., two families with teenagers work through an activity highlighting how family members hold different roles that are necessary and important when moving into different life stages).

Group members bring their unique experiences when completing an activity. In functional groups, individuals tend to work together to complete an initiative instead of forming separate alliances. It is beneficial for groups to be large enough to provide a diversity of ideas and abilities yet small enough so that individuals feel needed for the initiative's resolution. Groups also need to be small enough so that therapists can manage conflicts and model how to repair relationships after stabilizing the conflict.

Conducting group-based adventures also presents an opportunity to cultivate a supportive environment where group members can resolve conflict and practice communication in a culturally relevant manner. Group members adopt a systemic perspective as they struggle simultaneously to meet individual and group needs.

Potential learning conditions are directly and intentionally designed to arouse curiosity, strengthen client initiative and engagement, and create meaning in client investment. These group adventure factors combine to support the development of peer bonding, a strong growth of therapeutic alliance between therapist and client, group development, benefits from physical activity, and the clients' lives.

Challenging experiences

Challenge is the fourth mechanism through which adventure therapy supports transformation (Russell & Gillis, 2017). When properly implemented, adventure experiences introduce conditions that increase clients' motivation to change. The experiences foster these conditions through adaptive dissonance, natural consequences, synthesis/reflection, and active engagement in an activity. Adaptive dissonance occurs when clients adapt their behavior to resolve a conflict (dissonance). When clients work to resolve a conflict, they gain new skills and receive clear feedback from consequences that they can refer to in the future.

Adventure therapy strives to establish a climate of functional change through the positive use of eustress (i.e., positive use of stress). An experiential activity focuses on introducing eustress into the activity in a functional and manageable way (e.g., Selye, 1974). This type of stress places individuals into situations that activate positive problem-solving attributes (e.g., trust, cooperation, clear and healthy communication). Clients tend to also experience motivation due to the natural consequences inherent in the activities. Natural consequences are outcomes that occur without human intervention. Artificial consequences occur when the therapist or another person intervenes and provides feedback that may influence the person to modify their behavior.

Adventure experiences are often designed sequentially to allow clients to focus on challenges. As clients solve challenges, key outcomes such as competency, self-efficacy, and intrapersonal skills are heightened (Walsh & Golins, 1976). The incremental nature of adventure therapy allows clients to succeed at the tasks presented to them while gaining confidence and feeling empowered with new awareness, understanding, and skills related to their treatment goals. Adventure therapy ties well into the strength-based therapeutic approach, as activities are designed to be resolved successfully. Moreover, even if the activity is not completed "successfully" according to the intended goal, there are often ways to frame the experience as a success or as an opportunity for growth (e.g., clients who were minimally interacting are now taking on more responsibilities than earlier in the session).

Use of metaphor

The fifth mechanism, metaphor, is an enriching practice in many therapeutic approaches. It is a form of communication where an idea or object that ordinarily has a specific meaning in one context also possesses a figurative meaning in another. Milton Erickson (Haley, 1973) first applied metaphors instead of direct therapeutic suggestions to reduce client defenses and enhance therapeutic interventions. Minuchin (1981) and de Shazer (1982) found that metaphors offered powerful vehicles for therapeutic change when applied to therapeutic issues.

Another leader in the use of therapeutic metaphors was Bacon (1983, 1987). He provided a valuable bridge for the use of metaphors in adventure experiences. He stated four key components that must occur for the metaphor to be effective. The metaphor must: (1) be compelling enough to hold the individual's attention (e.g., related with appropriate intensity), (2) have a different successful resolution than the outcome in real life, (3) match the activity to treatment goals (i.e., isomorphic – "sameness of form"), and (4) be related in enough detail so that it will facilitate a client's transderivational search. Other therapists in psychotherapy who follow these elements in the creation and use of metaphors include de Shazer (1982), Haley (1988), Minuchin (1981), and Satir (1972/1990).

"Human Knot" is an example of how a metaphor could be incorporated into an adventure activity. After an introduction, the therapist explains the activity to a family of a heterosexual couple and four children aged 9–16 years. *"Today, we are starting in a circle, holding hands. To me, a circle represents a healthy family. Why do you think I say this?"* Participants give responses. *"What are ways that a circle does not represent a healthy family?"* Participants give responses. *"However, sometimes a family finds themselves not very happy. They may feel like they are all tied up like a knot, like your shoelaces. Now, I would like you to let go of your hands and reach across with your right hand to another person, not beside you. Awesome. Now, do the same thing with your left hand. This looks to me like a family who feels uncomfortable. This knot can be untangled using the skills we discussed in our last session and today about what a healthy family can look like. Do you have any questions before you begin?"*

Another example demonstrates how metaphors incorporated into an adventure therapy experience with youth can reveal qualities of client self-motivation and successful ending and promote kinesthetic-verbal responses. A youth with difficulty focusing on the details of school tasks participates in an adventure activity. The youth is asked to figure out the pathway through a maze by learning from the mistakes and successes of classmates, asking for help when unsure, practicing the pathway when others are trying, and taking appropriate risks.

Case study: Straight to your dreams

The following case example was created using an adventure therapy experience as a medium for change with an addicted, at-risk youth. In working with this youth and his family, I incorporated the following framework and adventure activity based on (1) the level of "isomorphism" (i. e., "same structure") where successful resolution of the adventure experience would assist in or lead to successful resolution of the therapeutic issue, and (2) the introduction of an experience that possessed an appropriate level of detail and emotion to stimulate a "transderivational" search in the client. (Note: There will be much more information on these two critical concepts in the following chapters).

The activity that was selected is commonly called the "Trust Lean" or "Willow in the Wind." It is probably most often used as a lead-up activity to the "Trust Fall," but it was an appropriate activity in this case. Note how the narrative is isomorphic with the father and son's experiences, and the adventure activity's resolution represents an outcome to the father and son's relationship. Note also that the narrative presented by the therapist is related in enough detail that it stimulates our client's transderivational search.

Goal

The therapeutic objective of this adventure experience was to re-direct inter-action between a father ("William") and a 14-year-old son ("Billy") who had become emotionally separated in a single-parent family. Presenting symptoms of the son's behavior included substance abuse, low self-esteem, and a strong fear that his father would also abandon him.

Sample presentation

"I'd like to do an exercise with the two of you to show you what I see as happening now in your family and how that will affect the future for both of you. This exercise is about (1) kids growing up to be adults, (2) how they figure out what they will be able to do and believe in themselves, and (3) testing limits.

Here, we have Billy facing away from the family and looking out into his future (position the son facing away). You're standing back here (place Dad behind son) supporting him like the good father that you are. In the exercise, Billy is moving forward toward his future, yet we all know that sometimes (and Billy has pointed this out to us), kids fall back and need to be repositioned. As you know, Dad, when this happens, you need to re-establish Billy's freedom as a growing boy while also keeping appropriate control as a parent. So, this exercise is about that; we know that all ado-lescents growing up will have setbacks, and parents are usually the best ones there to help their kids re-establish themselves and stay on the 'straight path.'

Before you enter this exercise of practicing the times that Billy will need your support, we'd better ensure that the two of you are there for each other. We'll do this with a series of statements that will proceed with Billy falling backward in this exercise. They will be:"

BILLY: "Are you there, Dad?"
DAD: "I'm here, Billy."

"Let's just try that." (Son and father go through statements. The thera-pist asks the son, *"When your father says that, are you sure that he's there?"* The son replies, *"No,"* and to punctuate this interaction, the therapist has the son turn around and go through the signals face-to-face with the father. The father is directed to assure the son that he will be there.)

"Now, Billy, your role here is to use your sensitivity and help your Dad the best you can. He wants all your future dreams to come true and for you to be the best person you can be, but he's also frightened for you. He doesn't know what he should let you do or where he should let you go. So, the best thing you can do to help him in this exercise is to show him that you trust him."

"In this exercise, like at other times, you don't just say trust; you show it. You show it here by staying straight. The straighter you are in this exercise, the more you show your Dad that you trust him and that he can trust you. So, stay straight in your ankles, knees, back, heart, neck, and head." (The therapist identifies each of these parts of the son as they are stated.) *"Staying straight with your body shows trust. If you really want to show him that you trust him and he can trust you, you will be as straight as possible, okay?"* (Son indicates he understands and agrees.)

THERAPIST: (to Dad) *"Now, there are several ways you can do your role here, Dad. You're a pretty strong guy, and you can stand back about 2– 3 feet, waiting for Billy to fall, or you can stay in touch with him throughout the process by starting from the very beginning of the exercise with your hands on his shoulders. Which do you think is best for you?"* (Father chooses to stand back and wait, which is consistent with his interaction with his son.)

"Okay, let's try it."

(Exercise is done with signals given first by the son and father. The son uneasily laughs at the signals and fails to lean back to his father. Son describes it as difficult for him to lean back on his father because he doesn't know if he's there or if his dad will catch him. The father changes his position to touch his son and reassure him that he is there.)

The therapist adds, *"I'm impressed with your change in your position and how much more comfortable Billy seems in this exercise. You know the more comfortable both of you get in Billy growing, the healthier the risks he can take will be. One thing we know is that if kids stand for nothing, they'll fall for anything, right?"*

"Another feature of this exercise is that it's one thing to give and cushion Billy in falling, but it's another to let him go too far. He could hit the floor or, worse yet, destroy his mind and body with things like drugs. Like all parents, you need to remember that you know what's best and appropriate for him."

Exercise is done again and accomplished where the father maintains contact with the son throughout the experience and re-positions the son after each setback. As the father demonstrates his competence in helping the son, the son's position in the exercise becomes totally straight.

2 Key principles of all effective therapies

While the specificity of presenting therapeutic issues differs with each client, key elements need to be adhered to and addressed to enhance the use of adventure therapy. This chapter outlines these critical foundational structures, including (a) understanding change concepts, (b) developing an appropriate therapeutic stance based on these concepts, (c) applying appropriate facilitation techniques, (d) establishing operating principles and ground rules, (e) listening effectively, (f) providing appropriate feedback, and (g) gathering critical information by observing client behaviors.

Understand the change concepts

Some initial concepts to understand why facilitation is important for adventure therapists include the principles, dynamics, and "rules" often associated with psychological change with clients. The following are concepts of change to consider, but certainly others can be added given the specific needs of clients:

1   There are no constant rules of change – As you can imagine, there are no rules of change that exist or occur all the time in therapy. Given this, it is important to examine the unique qualities of each circumstance with each specific client or client group. Efforts to impose inflexible facilitation and constant change practices run the risk of failure by not addressing or paying attention to the specifics of each situation.
2   Client assessment is critical – It is essential for adventure therapists to understand the specific conditions of each client's situation. Such details will always vary with each client, and addressing these variations is often critical to understanding client behavior in working with clients to produce healthy changes.
3   Types of change differ – Different types of change exist for clients. Bateson (1972) was one of the first therapists to recognize different change levels with clients in therapeutic situations. Understanding which method of change serves as the best path to achieve lasting

DOI: 10.4324/9781032640303-2

change for clients is key for adventure therapists. For example, first-order change centers on changing specific behaviors within the client's current system, whereas second-order change involves changing the very system of the client to change dysfunctional behaviors. Awareness of the most appropriate dynamics of change is a critical element of success with adventure therapy.

4   Create dissonance through eustress – The change process almost always disrupts existing behavior patterns with clients. As highlighted throughout the chapters in this book, adventure therapy fosters change by creating dissonance/challenges in clients' lives through the positive use of stress. It is the resolution of this dissonance that provides clients with integrative perspectives leading to changed behavior. Adventure therapists must create environments where clients feel supported in the very challenges that offer the dissonance to challenge their current behaviors and result in new, more functional behaviors.

5   Valuing changed behavior – Most change is rarely voluntary, and externally reinforced interventions are often ineffective, particularly with high client resistance. Clients behave in ways that make the most sense to them and often for reasons that appear to be their best alternative. Changing clients' behaviors should result in better alternatives for clients and some form of reward structure to make the change last.

6   Clients' best interests – Implementing change in clients' lives is an ethical decision. This can be especially true for clients who may not fully understand the ramifications/benefits of change. As clients enter adventure therapy programs, it is essential to establish programming principles connected with the client's long-term best interests.

7   Internalized change processes – For functional change behaviors to last, they must be internalized. This internalization process often depends upon the ability of program staff to provide experiences that will guide clients through this process. Experiential therapy experiences have several advantages over other therapeutic interventions because of the exciting, challenging, meaningful, memorable, and unique methods this process employs. Experiential therapists should use these advantages when creating connections to internalize change processes.

8   Client-centered change – Self-education is ultimately the best vehicle for clients to achieve lasting healthy change. Adventure therapists should focus on creating change experiences that help clients become aware of their dysfunction and, better yet, foster new, more functional, and beneficial behaviors.

Develop an appropriate therapeutic stance

As with all therapists, experiential therapy professionals must address several internal and external processes before appropriately assisting their clients. The four processes mentioned here certainly extend across all experiential therapy formats, and therapists are encouraged to add to this list for specific client issues and settings.

1   Understand your own personal belief system – Over time, all therapists will work with clients with differing belief systems, backgrounds, and cultural perspectives. The ability to effectively work with these different client groups depends on several factors, the first being the ability of the therapist to "know thyself." For example, if there are issues you cannot "join with" or remain neutral about with specific client systems, this affects your ability to assist the client. These are sometimes referred to as "non-negotiable values," or those beliefs you are unable or unwilling to support as an experiential therapist. Some common non-negotiable values for experiential therapists include violent behavior, sexist behavior, emotionally abusive language, physical abuse, etc. This does not mean you cannot work with clients with these issues, but you are unwilling to support these client behaviors in or as part of the therapeutic structure.

2   When you take inventory of your non-negotiable values before working with clients, you begin to learn what you can remain neutral and flexible about when issues arise. You will also be more prepared to deal with the value-laden concerns constantly occurring in therapeutic experiences.

3   Remain neutral to attain therapeutic mobility – Once your ability to identify non-negotiable values occurs, it becomes possible for you to take on a variety of "therapeutic stances" for client benefit. Such stances could include being a role model, a leader, a follower, a guide, etc. As Chapter 1 of this book outlines, one of the major strengths of adventure therapy is its role in serving as the central conduit of the experience, not the therapist. This "frees" the therapist to utilize greater flexibility/mobility to take on various roles that will serve the client best in their therapeutic process. Many therapists believe this ability to achieve and maintain a state of neutrality without being inappropriately distant from clients assists therapists in being more helpful in aiding their clients. Neutrality does not mean that "anything goes." On the contrary, it means the therapist can take on an appropriate strategic "position" that best serves the client during their therapeutic process. Such a stance places clients in charge of what they gain from an experience, and the therapist is freed to support clients in their efforts for change in a relevant and lasting manner.

4   Understand and clarify the role of the adventure therapist – From the beginning of the therapeutic process, the therapist needs to understand their role in the context of the client's background, current reality, and future state. Examples of this understanding and clarification include agreement on client diagnosis, how "success" will be viewed by the client and members of the client's "system," which responsibilities are the client's, and which are the therapist's, etc.

5   Proactively identify and operate from agreed-upon ethical principles and practices – Experiential therapists should conduct therapeutic practices from predetermined ethical principles and practices to protect clients and themselves. As seen in Appendix 1 of this book, the experiential therapy field has operated with evolving ethical principles in the areas of competence, integrity, responsibility, respect, concern, recognition, and objectivity since the early 1990s. These guidelines have been developed in conjunction with the Association for Experiential Education, and experiential therapists are encouraged to follow these ethical principles and address emerging and ongoing ethical dilemmas they encounter.

Apply appropriate facilitation concepts

The term most often used to describe the dialogue associated with the experiences is facilitation. In its simplest definition, facilitation means "to make it easier." And that is the role of adventure therapists in their clients' lives – to help co-construct therapeutic situations to make functional changes easier and more lasting for clients.

But why not just "tell" or dictate to clients what to do? Unfortunately, if this were the only thing necessary to produce functional change in clients' lives, most clients wouldn't need to participate in adventure therapy programs! Telling clients what to do, or what is healthier/more appropriate/more functional behavior, has usually already been attempted as a solution for most clients to deal with presenting problems or dysfunctional behaviors. Priest, Gass, and Gillis (2000, 2009) offer the following reasons why facilitation processes offer several advantages for adventure therapy:

- It generates greater "buy-in" or ownership in clients
- It provides a stronger focus on processes, generalized to future situations
- It increases access to the resolution of issues from a wide variety of sources
- It creates a greater possibility for the inclusion of multiple perspectives in problem-solving
- It places less dependence on adventure therapists to always provide the "right" answer for a particular issue
- It empowers clients to develop the best solutions for their issues
- It increases the construction of positive rapport and relationships among clients in therapeutic situations
- It seeks to utilize broad systemic perspectives on how positive changes can occur for clients
- It reinforces the building of a therapeutic environment that is open, positive, and involves high levels of client participation.

Establish appropriate conditions for change – Ground rules and operating principles

Critical to creating change in adventure experiences is establishing appropriate conditions for change. Such conditions are typically created in two ways: those established *externally for* the client by program staff and those created *internally by* clients (often facilitated by their adventure therapist). Ground rules are pre-established expectations created by adventure therapy staff for clients to follow during their adventure therapy experiences. Operating principles are created by clients representing the behavioral norms they want to use with one another in the adventure experience. Figure 2.1 contains examples of ground rules and operating principles designed at different times and for different purposes: (1) for the entire program, (2) during the therapeutic experience, and (3) in the therapeutic debriefing following adventure therapy experiences.

Note that establishing operating principles does not need to be a static or non-interactive experience. This activity itself can be quite experiential, often soliciting a higher degree of participant involvement with this active process. One common activity used to establish operating principles is the activity called "the Being" (Frank, 2001; Schoel & Maizell, 2002). The group uses a long (6') piece of butcher paper

Ground rules	Operating principles
Adventure therapist created	*Client created*
For the whole program	*For the whole program*
• Any form of violence is unacceptable • Agree/disagree with ideas, not people • No drugs	• Agree to focus on the present • Treat others like you want to be treated • Leave the past in the past
During the therapeutic experience	*During the therapeutic experience*

• You are responsible for your behavior
• You choose your level of participation
• You are responsible for the consequences
  of your actions
	• Everyone is expected to contribute
	• All rewards and consequences are shared
	  equally by group members
	• Work isn't done until everyone is finished

In the therapeutic debriefing session	*In the therapeutic debriefing session*
• Speak for yourself, not for others • Stay on the discussion topic • You have the right to pass on any topic	• One person speaks at a time • No interruptions • Listen carefully to others

Figure 2.1 Ground rules and operating principles for change

and felt tip markers in this activity. In most cases, the group traces the body of one person in their group onto the paper. Inside this outline, clients draw, sketch, or write behaviors that are important principles to follow as a group. On the outside of this outline, they draw, sketch, or write behaviors that are important *not* to occur in group interactions. This paper is generally posted in a visible area and referred to as the group begins therapeutic interactions. Adaptations to these new operating principles are recorded on the paper as the group progresses through adventure therapy experiences.

The more clients can create operating principles instead of relying on adventure therapists to develop ground rules, the healthier/more functional the therapeutic group. Adventure therapists are also encouraged to clearly word the commitments in these behavioral contracts. The clearer the expected behaviors and established norms are, the less likely future misunderstandings will occur.

Listen effectively

Encouraging clients to communicate, listen to what they say, and comprehend what they are trying to convey are critical when facilitating client growth. Facilitating change is only possible if these requisite factors of communication exist. Priest, Gass, and Gillis (2000, 2009) offered these ten effective listening guidelines for adventure therapists to use when culturally and clinically appropriate:

- Maintain appropriate eye contact with clients (e.g., lean forward to invite disclosure).
- Signal your attentiveness with verbal and nonverbal affirmation (e.g., saying "yes" while nodding your head).
- Wait through pauses to encourage clients to resume talking; don't rush to fill in silences and be patient.
- Use open-ended questions to encourage clients to continue talking or to probe for deeper collaboration (e.g., "What do you mean by that?" or "Please tell us more about this").
- Summarize and paraphrase clients' remarks to demonstrate your comprehension of their ideas.
- Respond to feelings that may lie behind clients' words by showing empathy for how they feel.
- Use a gentle tone of voice expressing care rather than judgment.
- Listen for action words (i.e., verbs ending in "ing") depicting a process rather than a product orientation.
- Separate behaviors clients identify as unchangeable from those appearing to be changeable, particularly by the client.
- Don't take the focus of the conversation away from clients by changing the subject or by agreeing or disagreeing. Stay on the subject area

by simply indicating the message was understood and use neutral comments like "that's interesting" rather than good or bad value-laden labels.

Listening is a therapeutic skill that needs to be constantly practiced and evaluated. Seeking feedback from other adventure therapists about what they do to enhance their listening skills is a worthwhile practice.

Provide appropriate feedback

Another critical skill of adventure therapists is the ability to provide appropriate feedback to clients. Feedback is the exchange of verbal and nonverbal messages between therapists and clients, as well as clients among themselves when in group processing. For feedback to be valuable, it needs to follow certain guidelines. Feedback tends to be most effective when it describes demonstrated behaviors, refers to specific behaviors, is presented with positive intention, is directed toward something the recipient can change, is sought out by the receiver, is delivered when it can be best understood, is verified/validated by the recipient, and can be double-checked with other supportive and well-intentioned group members for accuracy. Feedback tends to be less effective when it is done for evaluation purposes only, is expressed in general terms, is meant to "put down" or be destructive to the recipient, is not sought out by the recipient but delivered anyway, is offered at a bad time, is not double-checked with the recipient, and ignores potential input from other group members. Figure 2.2 outlines eight characteristics of appropriate feedback adventure therapists should seek to follow (Priest, Gass, & Gillis, 2009).

Gather critical information by observing client behaviors

Adventure therapists gather a great deal of information from what clients say and what they see clients do. In Chapter 1, this was referred to as one of the adventure therapy approach's strengths – the ability to examine clients' "walk as well as talk." To take advantage of this critical aspect of adventure therapy, adventure therapists are encouraged to be vigilant in these two aspects. Figure 2.3 outlines one method of monitoring what is said (i.e., verbal) as well as what is done (i.e., nonverbal) in adventure therapy experiences (Priest, Gass, & Gillis, 2009).

Feedback is ...	Feedback is not...	Explanation
Descriptive	Evaluative	Descriptive feedback offers observations, not assessing the value of what clients have done. This produces defensive or resistant behavior.
Specific	General	Specific feedback lessens misinterpretation and provides substance for clients to examine and potentially learn from.
Well-intended	Destructive	Focus feedback intentions on producing client-centered functional behavior.
Directed toward change	Directed toward something that can't be changed	Provide feedback only about behaviors clients can change and learn from.
Solicited	Imposed	Feedback is most useful when clients seek and value it. Provide the appropriate manner and forum for presenting feedback to clients.
Well-timed	Inappropriately presented	Present feedback at the appropriate times and with enough time to fully complete what needs to be said.
Verified with the recipient	Not verified with the recipient	Periodically check in with clients to see if your message and intention of feedback is the same as what they understand.
Verified with the group	Ignores the group	When working with groups, use other clients to provide a sounding board for feedback. This can add consistency as well as variations to client behavior.

Figure 2.2 Key principles of all effective therapies

Clue	Verbal	Nonverbal
Who?	Who speaks to whom? Who speaks for others?	Who makes eye contact with you or others? Who avoids looking at people?
What?	What is the discussion topic? What is NOT discussed?	What are clients doing during discussion? What are clients doing when NOT speaking?
When?	Is the topic of discussion timely? When do people avoid the topic?	When are clients ready to change? When are clients resistant to change?
Where?	Where is the direction of the discussion going?	Where do clients stand on issues? Where do clients exert their influence on topics?
How?	How do group members attempt to shift the discussion topic?	How do clients treat one another? How do clients interact during conflict?

Figure 2.3 Verbal and nonverbal cues for feedback

3 Adventure therapy assessment

Assessments in behavioral healthcare settings are the processes used to collect constructive information on client's issues. Interventions are typically seen as the processes professionals implement to address those issues uncovered by client assessment. As illustrated by the quotation at the beginning of this chapter, these concepts are inextricably linked. The best assessments by a clinician lead to implementing accurate interventions, and such interventions will typically provide the richest resources for future assessments.

As early as 1983, therapists started to formally recognize the assessment qualities of adventure experiences. In Kimball's (1983) work with clients in institutional and clinical settings, he found that traditional clinical assessment procedures sometimes failed to provide a complete and accurate assessment of clients' needs and issues. Some reasons for these failures included: (1) the information gathered from written paper and pen assessments covered reported behaviors but not observed and validated ones, and (2) on assessment procedures, clients responded with "social self" responses rather than "true self" responses (i.e., clients provided answers the testers were looking for or that would be rewarded, rather than what the "right answers" were). The outcomes found in adventure experiences created an environment where accurate appraisals of client issues could be obtained using adventure experiences as psychological projective tools. By carefully observing key client responses to specific adventure experiences, therapists can identify critical behavior patterns, dysfunctional behaviors, coping mechanisms, and responses. One key difference between adventure therapy experiences and traditional assessments taken in a clinician's office is that there was no way to "fake" one's way through the adventure experience because of the unfamiliarity with what was expected or valued by the clinician (i.e., "the body does not know how to lie").

The assessment model illustrated here combines the CHANGES model (Gass & Gillis, 1995) and the GRABBSS model (Schoel & Maizell, 2002). The CHANGES model covers clients' macro assessment or systemic issues, while the GRABBSS model addresses the change process's micro assessment or individual perspectives.

DOI: 10.4324/9781032640303-3

Macroassessment: CHANGES

The CHANGES model is a six-step interactive yet differentiated process used before, during, and after the therapeutic experience (see Figure 3.1). The CH (or CHEW) part of the model primarily assesses the current context of clients and their issues, building tentative hypotheses to be tested and examining how issues present themselves. The ANG part of the model leads the therapist to utilize the novelty of adventure experiences to help generate processes of the clients' reality. And the ES integrates important cues in identifying and evaluating potential outcomes and solutions for the clients and their issues. The following discussion offers a fuller explanation of these steps and a case study that further illustrates these concepts.

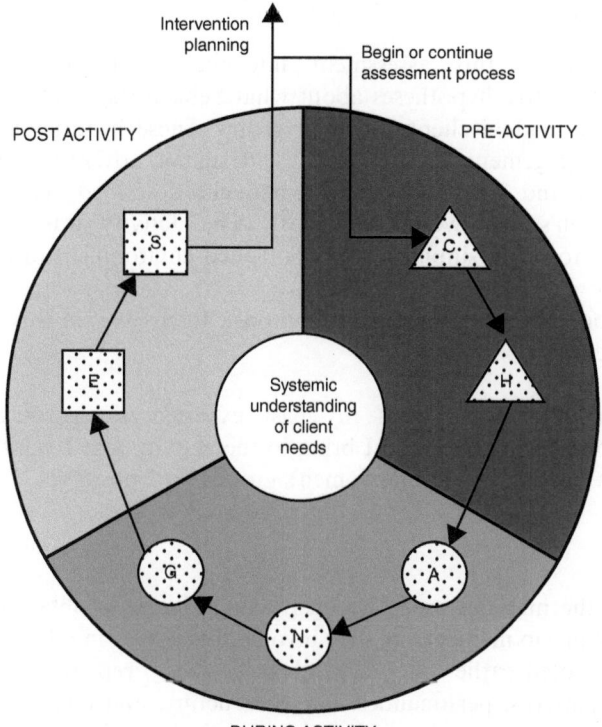

Figure 3.1 The CHANGES model (Gass & Gillis, 1995) is a helpful way to organize interaction to acquire information and reflect upon it to develop functional client change. The seven steps that make up the acronym CHANGES are Context, Hypotheses, Action, Novelty, Generating, Evaluation, and Solutions

Context

Information provides context. In clinical settings, individual client information that is gathered at intake can be assessed as treatment progresses (e.g., progress monitoring) and later used as pre-post indicators of changes in psychosocial outcomes attributed to the AT experience.

Questions therapists might ask in this part of the model include:

- Where am I working and with whom (e.g., cis-gendered males or females, coed or single sex, transgender or nonbinary, adults or adolescents, substance users, trauma survivors)?
- Am I competent, and can I be competent, with this group given the parameters of the situation (e.g., do these factors set me up for success or failure)?

Hypotheses

After gathering this assessment information, adventure therapists establish tentative hypotheses about what behavior(s) might be expected from the individual client and their group. These hypotheses are tested through engagement in intentionally designed adventure experiences. The "Walk and Talk" adventure experience described below was used in a women's empowerment activity. The activity was intentionally structured to begin similar to the controlled environment of a treatment program.

Questions adventure therapists might ask themselves in this part of the model include:

- What information from my past experiences regarding womens' empowerment groups do I bring to the activity that I want to test?
- What information about women's groups do I possess?

Action

Much of the material used for constructing change is obtained from the actions of group members as they involve themselves in adventure experiences. As noted earlier, group members project a representation of their behavior patterns, personalities, family structure, and interpretation onto the adventure activities because they are typically unfamiliar with what is being asked of them in the experience. The adventure therapist in the case discussed here was able to observe how individual group members utilized resilience techniques to handle substance use issues.

Questions adventure therapists might ask themselves in this part of the model include:

- Are clients' actions congruent or incongruent with your hypotheses?
- Do initial hypotheses confirm, adapt, revise, or reject your thoughts?
- Can you engage clients in their motivational areas, not your own?

Novelty

Actions that are unfamiliar or new to the group can result in group members needing help with the spontaneity of an adventure experience. As a result, group members do not always know how they are expected to act, which prevents them from hiding behind a false or "social" self. This further leads them to show their true behaviors and provides additional information to the adventure therapist. Karl Rohnke (1988, personal communication) has often commented that when you bring out a basketball or soccer ball, most youth have expectations of what might follow. These expectations can be positive or negative, depending on past experience. However, bringing out a pool noodle or a rubber chicken usually does not engender assumptions of what might happen next. The result can be a heightened sense of projection.

In this part of the model, adventure therapists might consider including the following:

- The strong use of spontaneity, which allows therapists to see the real/core issues of the client group instead of the "socially proper" ones because of the spontaneous manner the clients use to respond.
- The strong use of projection, as people typically do not come to the experience with preconceived ideas of success or failure (e.g., how they are supposed to act) because they have no previous knowledge base to determine socially accepted roles.

Generating

By carefully observing group members' responses to a multitude of actions, adventure therapists can identify functional and dysfunctional behaviors; concrete, abstract, distorted, or critical thinking patterns; and appropriate or inappropriate affect. These patterns are most accurately perceived when a functional relationship (therapeutic alliance) exists between an adventure therapist and the client or client group.

Questions adventure therapists might ask themselves in this part of the model include:

- What is the clients' language (e.g., are there words with isomorphic connections or homonyms)?
- What are the clients' value systems and beliefs?

- Can you track behavior patterns (e.g., what happens in what order)?
- What are the cyclical patterns of behavior?
- How can the therapist understand why, and at what level, this behavior makes sense?
- Is there a congruency between actions and spoken words?
- What is the interplay of intimacy, closeness, distance, boundaries, etc.?
- Are group member roles assumed alliances, or are they "at odds" over particular issues?
- What communication techniques are used (e.g., nonverbal/verbal, speaking through another person)?
- What is the therapist's intuition saying about what is going on?

Evaluation

When information has been generated from observations of the group's behaviors, it can be compared with the working hypotheses once again. Do group actions fit the working hypotheses? Are these hypotheses supported or refuted? What new knowledge now exists to revisit action, novelty, and generating in the next experience?

Questions adventure therapists might ask themselves in this part of the model include:

- What are the therapists' interpretations of the information generated by the client group?
- What type of general, specific, and circular feedback is occurring?
- Which hypotheses are being confirmed or rejected?
- Which hypotheses seem to be validated by client behavior?

Solutions

Finally, and most importantly, when the evaluation provides a clear picture of the group's issues, it can lead to solutions. Integrating and interpreting the information gathered in previous steps helps therapists decide how to construct potential solutions to the group's concerns. Although these solutions can be reached within one session, it is more likely that (over the history of this particular group) the activities and actions that worked well would be increased, thus potentially pushing out negative actions to lead to a healthier group.

Questions adventure therapists might ask themselves in this part of the model include:

- What would be potential solutions to the issues?
- If problems are noted, are there exceptions when they do not exist?

- How can clients do more of what is working in order to resolve their issues?

It has become evident that for clinicians to use adventure experiences as assessment tools properly, they must possess an awareness of potential structures or archetypes that reside within the preexisting contexts of both the adventure experience and common actions. To ascribe some sense of meaning to client actions, clinicians must be aware of how their clients interpret these structures or archetypes. This is where adventure experiences are similar to Rorschach testing, where clients project interpretation on an unknown structured drawing. But where adventure experiences differ is in the motivating factor of movement and the dynamic, multi-dimensional, and parallel structures that exist in actions rather than just on a piece of paper.

Case study: Walk the Talk

This metaphorical activity was developed for a relapse prevention group in Singapore. The activity was designed for the last 45 minutes of a three-hour relapse group meeting. One of the reasons I like the title of this activity (and introduce the experience using this name) is that it has a great connection to what the group members will face once they leave the therapy room.

All group members presented a history of substance use and were in various stages of their recovery process. The following case history examples of three group members are provided to give an idea of the sample client background.

Chin S. became involved with drugs after serving his National Service at the age of 17. He was working as a sales representative and was introduced to heroin by a colleague. He was apprehended by the Central Narcotics Bureau (CNB) about one year after he started using heroin. He also had tried other drugs such as ganja and ketamine.

Chin S. was sent to a DRC and underwent rehabilitation/treatment and was released 18 months later. After his release, Chin S. was assigned to a Volunteer Aftercare Officer (VAO) who worked with Chin S. on his recovery issues and helped him start his life anew and find employment. He acknowledges that staying away from old colleagues is key to his recovery process.

Malek had been introduced to drugs by friends, starting with glue-sniffing, ganja, pills, and then heroin. He was arrested for use at 26 and released one year later. He began mixing with his addict friends again and returned to his old drug habits. He was rearrested again eight months later. Malek's wife and son visited him at the DRC. Upon release, he was assigned to an Aftercare Case Manager (ACM) and reports regularly for CNB supervision.

Mala grew up in a family of people with addiction. She had been exposed to drugs at a young age, her father had a heroin addiction for more than 20 years, and her three brothers used drugs and sometimes physically abused her (e.g., slapping and hitting her so they could get her money). Mala developed a relationship with a man from her workplace, and he introduced her to drugs. The CNB raided her boyfriend's house when they were smoking, and both were sent to a DRC for rehabilitation/ treatment. During counseling, she expressed regret and shared how much pressure she faced to use drugs from her boyfriend. She wanted to turn over a new leaf when released.

When released, Mala turned back to her family. Her brothers returned to their "physical abuse for money" pattern. One day, returning from work, a friend of Mala's encouraged her to take a straw to relax. Mala initially rejected her, but she took it after much persuasion. Before long, Mala began smoking again and got trapped in her addictive cycle. After about three months, she was caught again and sent to a DRC.

The relapse group consisted of 12–15 clients (ages 20–35) with histories of drug abuse. They were in various stages of the recovery process, trying to maintain a drug-free lifestyle, often under challenging conditions. A common theme in their lives was the temptation to return to a drug-using lifestyle (often from friends and family members), even though they possessed a sincere desire to stay drug-free and a strong knowledge of the consequences that returning to using would have on their lives.

Goals

The experience, presented in this manner, emphasizes: (1) maintaining a drug-free lifestyle; (2) identifying, staying connected to, and having a strong focus on the elements of maintaining abstinence; and (3) strengthening clients' resistance to the social temptations that often occur to try and get them to begin using again.

Set-up

The adventure experience used for these treatment objectives is the "Stepping Stones" activity (e.g., see Rohnke & Butler, 1995, pp. 186–188). The equipment needed is (1) two ropes to mark the "beginning" and "finish" lines; (2) a flat, unobstructed distance of anywhere from 20 to 50 meters; and (3) one large paper plate per person that can be written on (4) markers.

The goal is to get from one end line to the other without touching the ground between the beginning and end lines. People are positioned behind the beginning line and provided with approximately 25 minutes to get over the finish line.

Anyone touching the ground between the lines must return to the beginning. At ANY TIME during the experience, if anyone loses physical contact with any prop, the group loses that prop to the facilitator (NOTE: THIS IS A KEY RULE).

Note you can use the rule that props can only move forward, or they can also move backward or forward. Either dynamic will set up different issues. The "bad part" about letting props go backward is that people often get creative: one person might grab two props, "skate" across the gap, and somehow return the props to the start for others to do the same thing. This can undermine the whole purpose of the activity.

The "good part" of this dynamic is that it facilitates the idea that they can move backward, since that has a nice isomorphic connection to the temptation a lot of people with an addiction feel toward helping friends with their issues, often at the risk of jeopardizing their own recovery.

Here's what I would suggest. Don't announce this as a beginning rule. If people initially start to use this as a strategy, fall back on the old excuse of "facilitator brain lock" and tell them they can't do this. If they don't do this immediately and start to lose a substantial number of props (e.g., more than five), permit it to happen. If you decide to let props go back, only one prop can be returned at a time.

For physical considerations, note there is no running or jumping (this is hard to do anyway in this experience). No throwing of props. People cannot climb on each other's backs.

For emotional considerations, the more serious clients are about staying abstinent from drugs, the better the activity. Clients must be ready to face the symbolic messages in the activity associated with making bad decisions. It is important to allow time to process the experience following the activity.

Sample presentation

(Presentation stated in a group circle where everyone can see each other and the counselor.)

COUNSELOR: *"It's been good to be together for the last couple of hours and share your triumphs and concerns about your recovery process. And even though we've addressed some hard topics, it is almost too comfortable here in this room! I say this because while it's tough looking at the things we've addressed today, it will almost certainly be tougher for all of you when you step through the door of this room at the end of our group meeting. You know it is not a matter of IF you will be tempted to use drugs again, but WHEN you will face this decision again. And this decision will not come from strangers but often from people you know best and who may be close to you.*

One of the great things we have gone over here are the qualities, commitments, and elements you feel will help you stay drug-free. And in our discussions, it seems the more committed and connected you stay to these elements or qualities, the more likely you are to make it back into this room drug-free next week.

And this is what the final activity of our time here today is all about. It's about (1) how to make it back here to this meeting next week drug-free, (2) how to stay connected to those things helping you maintain your abstinence, and (3) how to strengthen your resistance to the temptations that will occur, trying to get you to use drugs again.

But before we begin, I want you to each take a plate and write on the back of it one to three words describing a quality or phrase you think will help you stay drug-free over the next week, particularly one that if you stay connected to and focused on it, it will help you to remain drug-free. After you've done this, let's go around the circle and have each person share what they've written and briefly describe why they feel staying connected to and focused on this quality is so important."

*(*After everyone has shared their quality) *"Okay, please join me over here on this flat stretch of ground behind this line. Here's the way I see it, and you might see it this way too. Behind this line represents us right now in this room. Confronting in some ways, but in others, it's safe and comfortable. The thing is, we can't stay in this room here forever! In 45 minutes or so, we are all going to walk out that door and be in places over the next week that are going to challenge our abilities to stay drug-free. And there is probably no better time than now to start practicing for those times. After explaining the rules of the activity, I will give you five to seven minutes to plan and talk as a group about how you might want to consider going about this process.*

Here's the deal: you need to get from this line here over across that line 30 meters away, just like you need to get from where you are here today once you leave, back to this meeting room next week. As you go from line to line, you must not touch the ground. If you do, you need to return to the beginning of this line. The only way you can do this is by using your qualities (i.e., plates) as protection to step on to get across to the other line. If your foot remains on your plate and no other part of your body touches the (e.g., arm), you're fine.

You also must stay in constant contact with your resources. If at ANY TIME you lose connection with your plate, even for a split second, I (representing addiction) will get to take it from you.

You have 25 minutes to get over the end line. Again, anyone touching the ground between the ropes must return to the beginning. At ANY TIME OR INSTANT, if a person loses physical contact with any resource, the group loses that prop to me. If there are no questions, your five minutes of planning begins. Good luck."

Logistics

Care needs to be taken to clarify rules, punctuate isomorphic connections of the activity to clients' recovery processes, and watch carefully for people losing contact with their plates/resources. Planning can occur long after their initial five to seven-minute period is completed; it's just that their 25 minutes of activity time begins after their plan time expires.

Losing contact often happens at very innocent times when people lift a foot, go to place a plate down, or just simply aren't paying attention (which may have some strong relation to issues that are going to arise over the coming week). If clients decide to return to try and help others, punctuating the consequences of their decisions may provide rich insight into dynamics such as enabling, boundary issues, enmeshment, etc.

Debriefing

Debriefing focuses on the three therapeutic objectives of the activity and how they relate to the clients' coming week. As clients leave I sometimes anchor individual learnings for each participant with selected words and appropriate physical connection (e.g., handshake, squeeze on the shoulder).

4 Adventure therapy metaphors

A single word can possess multiple meanings;
but as the common saying goes, a picture can be worth 1000 words.
And if a picture can be worth 1000 words,
And if an experience can be worth 1000 pictures,
then one metaphor can be worth 1000 experiences.
But a metaphor possesses its greatest worth; when it
interprets the right experience that
provides the right picture that
produces the words that
have relevant meaning for a person.

(Gass, 1991)

One of the primary goals of an adventure therapist is to foster the development of lasting functional change for clients through adventure experiences. Metaphors are frequently used by adventure therapists to reach this common objective. Metaphors are generally defined as a form of communication where an idea or object that ordinarily has a specific and literal meaning on one level also possesses the likeliness and figurative meaning on another level. Metaphors obtain their richness, as well as their complexity or confusion, in the process of human communication.

Several of the reasons for using metaphors with clients in adventure therapy include:

1   Metaphors can make the treatment experience more inductive and relevant for clients. When an appropriate metaphoric framework is properly utilized it connects the adventure experience to the clients' lives in a way where the successful resolution of the adventure experience provides a pathway, structure, or guidance in reaching their intended therapeutic objective.
2   Kinesthetic elements of therapy (i.e., "messages in the movement") are used in conjunction with cognitive behavioral principles to increase the likelihood of achieving therapeutic objectives.
3   Metaphors utilize conscious learning patterns that help to promote access to the unconscious mind. They recognize relevant structure/patterns, often

DOI: 10.4324/9781032640303-4

through transderivational search patterns. Several researchers (e.g., Doherty, 1995; Gass & Priest, 2006) have found that properly structured metaphors with adventure experiences not only can produce greater client gains, but also maintain growth for longer periods of time.

To see how the mind creates mental structures or patterns that affect our thinking and actions, quickly read out loud the following four sentences and fill in the blank with the final word:

> *To stick someone with a pole is called a "poke,"*
> *to tell a funny story to make you laugh is called a "joke,"*
> *the tree that drops acorns is called an "oak,"*
> *and the white part of a boiled egg is called a "_____."*

The final word people place in the blank above is generally "yolk," when it should be "egg white." But a few associated factors (e.g., the answer is a single syllable word, each sentence fragment ends with a word that rhymes with "folk," and the consistent agreement regarding the definite articles of "a" and "an") frame the response to be "incorrect."

4   Metaphors stimulate associational memory (i.e., the process of making connections between experiences in a unique and simultaneous way) (Hager, 2008).
5   Metaphors used by other forms of psychotherapy (e.g., de Shazer, 1982; Haley, 1988; Minuchin, 1981; Satir, 1972/1990) do not possess kinesthetic elements that are the basis of adventure therapy experiences.
6   This is often done by bypassing learned limitations and negative beliefs because they are so rich in information the conscious mind is unable to filter out and ends up unable to handle all the information it's receiving. Let's look at an example of this. When metaphors are used to stimulate a transderivational search, the unconscious part of the mind is accessed to interpret the contextual understandings and areas of growth.

Let's look at an example of how the unconscious part of the brain can work. The first thing you need to do is remain on this page until you have read and understood the directions below.

Instructions: After you have read these directions, you will turn the page and read for ONLY (2) seconds and no more. You will then be asked about what you saw.

Are you ready? Remember, 2 seconds only!

Pillow Slumber Dream
Bed Tired Exhausted
Quiet Nap Snore

Thinking back at what you saw on the previous page, what words did you read? Was the word "sleep" on the page? From a literal or conscience perspective, "sleep" was not on the page. But from a subconscious, metaphorical, or association perspective, the word "sleep" may have been on your list.

Kinesthetic metaphors

The use of metaphoric structures has been outlined by several individuals outside of the field of adventure therapy. Probably the individual credited most often with the development of therapeutic metaphor is Milton Erickson. In his work, Erickson (Rossi, 1980; Haley, 1973) found that using metaphors instead of direct therapeutic suggestions reduced clients' defenses and enhanced therapeutic interventions. Minuchin (1981) and de Shazer (1982) also stated that when metaphors contained linking "isomorphs" (i.e., possessed "equivalent structures") to therapeutic issues, they offered powerful vehicles for therapeutic change. Isomorphism, a concept initially developed by scientists and mathematicians (Hofstadter, 1979), occurs when two complex structures of different situations can be mapped on to one another so that similar features can be linked together. Once the connection of these features is made, the similar roles they play in their respective structures creates a medium for change. This medium provides possible connections for the transfer of valuable information learned in one environment for use in another.

Bacon (1983, 1987) provided a valuable bridge for the use of metaphors in the development of adventure therapy experiences. In creating such experiences, he stated that four key components must occur for the metaphor to be effective. The metaphor must: (1) be compelling enough to hold the individual's attention (i.e., it must be related with appropriate intensity), (2) have a different successful ending/resolution from the corresponding real-life experience, (3) be isomorphic, (4) be related in enough detail that they can facilitate a student's "transderivational search" (i.e., a process first described by Carl Jung where the client attaches personal meaning to archetypical experiences). Bacon stated that when these four conditions are met, adventure experiences provide more successful resolutions to formally unproductive and dysfunctional behaviors, creating opportunities for positive therapeutic change within clients (Bacon, 1987). Gass (1986, 1990) furthered this development of metaphor in adventure experiences, pointing to the belief that resolution of adventure experiences can lead to successful resolution of client issues.

Metaphoric transfer

Trust Fall (aka Fall from Height) Initiative at a drug treatment program:

THERAPIST: *"Probably lots of you think that this initiative has something to do with trusting others, or with knowing that people will support you if you let them. And that's a fine meaning to get out of this activity. But our purpose in choosing this exercise is different; we picked it because it may possess an even more important lesson here. And that lesson concerns letting go of your old lifestyle. Let me tell you a bit more about what I mean.*

Each of you will be getting up here and holding on to this tree before falling backwards. Before you fall, I'm going to ask you to close your eyes and imagine that the tree is that part of your personality – that piece of you – most responsible for your drinking and drugging. I don't want you to think of this as a tree anymore; I want you to think of it as the most powerful factor responsible for your using. And I want you to hug it like you love it – like it's all you've got.

Because after you hold on to it for, for 30 seconds; I'm going to ask you to let go – to give up and let go of whatever it is that keeps you drinking and drugging. You'll just lie back and fall towards these people.

And don't be surprised if you feel a little nervous. All alcoholics/ addicts have at least some love for their old lifestyle, no matter how much they really want to change it. And there's always some degree of hesitation towards committing to a drug-free life. Cause you don't know what it is like. So, I'd be surprised if you didn't feel some kind of nervousness about falling."

(Bacon, 1991, pp. 11–12)

Metaphoric transfer can occur in three ways (Bacon & Kimball, 1989):

1   placing a client in situations as a parallel: isomorphic (i.e., "same structure") connections occur *spontaneously* between the adventure experience and the therapeutic objective,
2   having a client participate in adventure experiences first and then reflect on the *analogous* metaphoric connections between the adventure experience and their therapeutic issues, or
3   proactively and appropriately "frame" or structure each metaphoric experience to directly induct a client into integrating functional changes into their lives. Appropriate framing can enhance the value of the adventure therapy experience, enabling it to be more prescriptive and specific in its application and use. The proper structuring of metaphoric adventure activities often holds the key to creating effective experiences and lasting change for clients.

While all three of the types of metaphoric transfer listed previously – spontaneous metaphoric transfer, analogous metaphoric transfer, and structured metaphoric transfer (Bacon & Kimball, 1989) – can be found in the adventure therapy field, it is increasingly evident from research (Doherty, 1995, Gass & Priest, 2006), case studies (Gass & Dobkin, 1991; Gass,

1995), and theory (Bacon, 1983; Gass, 1991) that adventure therapy professionals need to develop appropriate expertise to successfully structure metaphoric experiences.

For example, take the presenting problem of attention deficit hyperactivity disorder. The DSM-5-TR (American Psychiatric Association, 2022) lists the presenting behaviors of ADHD as:

- difficulty *paying attention* to details and tendency to *make careless mistakes* in school or other activities, producing work that is often messy and careless
- easily *distracted by irrelevant stimuli* and frequently interrupting ongoing tasks to attend to trivial noises or events that are usually ignored by others
- *inability to sustain attention* on tasks or activities
- *difficulty finishing* schoolwork or paperwork or *performing tasks that require concentration*
- *frequent shifts* from one uncompleted activity to another
- *forgetfulness* in daily activities (e.g., missing appointments, forgetting lunch)
- frequent shifts in conversation, not listening to others, not keeping one's mind in conversations, and *not following details or rules* of activities in social situations.

Nested within these presenting symptoms are the very clues for what activities might be selected for use with this population. Notice the phrases in italics (e.g., *difficulty paying attention, distracted by irrelevant stimuli, inability to sustain attention, difficulty finishing, frequent shifts, forgetfulness, not following details or rules*). An adventure therapist takes these clues, frames them in terms of selecting functional behaviors to address these issues, and selects adventure experiences that promote healthy and functional behavior. In this case, the kinesthetic metaphor would be composed of experiences centered on focused attention, remembering, listening, etc.; those very activities that promote functional behavior. Two adventure experiences directly selected to address the presenting ADHD issues listed above can be seen at the websites of videos below:

AEE09 ADHD activity: https://www.youtube.com/watch?v=kD98FjdnJEQ. AEE09 hands follow pattern: http://www.youtube.com/watch?v=1uS1Nyrx87U&feature=related.

Each of these structured kinesthetic metaphor experiences addresses key issues associated with ADHD and rewards functional behavior in the experience for the various clients. This kinesthetic involvement with the client makes the therapeutic use of metaphor richer and more influential. More information on the structured use of kinesthetic metaphors in adventure therapy metaphors can be found at the following website: http://kinestheticmetaphors.com/AEE_ 2009.html.

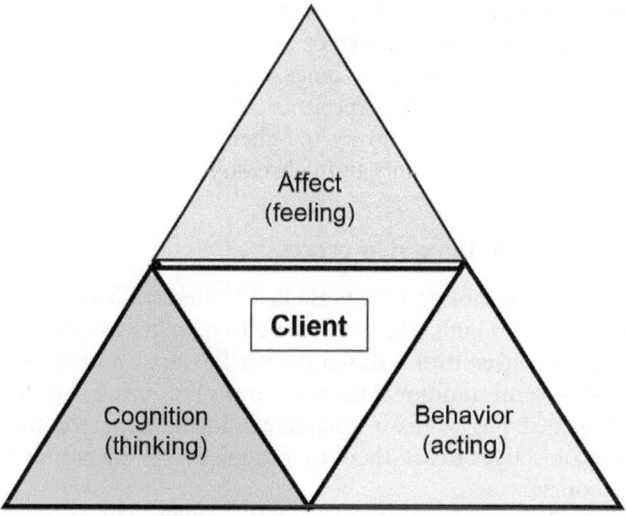

Figure 4.1 An integrative ABC model for adventure therapy settings

Isomorphically framing the experience

Gass, Gillis, and Russell (2020) introduced the ABC/R triangle as a visual representation of how adventure therapists can join and intervene with clients (Figure 4.1). The "A" of this model stands for affect, the "B" stands for behavior, the "C" stands for cognition, and the "R" for relationship. When working with clients, adventure therapists focus on engaging clients in feelings (affect), actions (behavior), and cognition (thinking). The therapist considers the therapeutic treatment plan and decides which aspect should be emphasized during the activity. Maybe a client is having challenges with communicating their feelings so the activity could focus more on that affective aspect than the behavior or cognition.

Developing structured metaphors: A three step process

This section will outline how adventure therapists make these connections using kinesthetic metaphors. When properly using this approach, the client can attain deeper levels of understanding. The didactic and verbal processes of traditional therapies are augmented in adventure experiences through concrete kinesthetic experiences. Clients' behaviors are viewed from differing perspectives as they are asked to "walk and talk" rather than merely "talk" their behaviors.

This three-step model consists of: (1) matching the client's narrative to a metaphor that is isomorphic to the client's issue, (2) moving out of the chair/couch and conduct a novel adventure yet isomorphic experience, and

(3) positioning and conducting the client in the experience so a successful resolution of the adventure experience results in strengthening functional change. Note that there are two times when transderivational searches occur during the therapeutic experience. One occurs by the therapist during the first step. The second by the client during the second to third step when the client is reflecting and debriefing.

Case study using the three step process

I was working with a mother who presented feelings of being overwhelmed in "handling" her two boys. She wanted me to help her use strategies to get her two boys "under control." Based on her life story and associated language through several traditional family therapy sessions, I believed she and her Sons provided me with an adequate understanding of their family structure and objectives to ask them to join me for an adventure activity at a challenge course.

The Incline Log initiative (e.g., Rohnke, 1989; Webster, 1988) was framed with the two guiding treatment objectives: (1) focus on the language they used between each other (e.g., supportive and working together language) and (2) select an experience rich in potential connections to this client's life story. The goal of the activity was to walk up a slanted log while being belayed with a rope by someone significant. When the Son was walking the log, his Mother was holding the rope that kept him safe. I encouraged her Son to communicate to her on what he needed to reach his goal (i.e., the top). The dialogue centered around her Son asking for "slack" (the Mom making the rope to her Son not be too tight) when he was doing well and moving (e.g., independent, being trusted) and then calling "Up rope" when he felt like he might fall (e.g., his need to have some help, Mom's desire to "reign" him in, give guidance, set boundaries). I also encouraged her to have fun and explore how she could support and reinforce him in reaching his goal.

During the experience, I also encouraged her Son to communicate with his Mother on what he needed to reach his goal, making observations during the activity that when his messages came through clearly, he usually received the "slack" from his Mom he wanted as opposed to when he was misunderstood.

During our reflection after the experience, as well as in another "sit-down" therapy session, our dialogue centered around highlighting the learnings from the experience. Several areas were discussed and included:

1   The relationship of Mom providing "slack" to her Son when he was successful and how this success tended to continue when she recognized positive effort and provided support.
2   How when Mom gave her Son some "slack," he was able to go up the incline log much easier and progress, versus when she held him back

(inappropriately) he became "stuck." Our discussion further centered around the family's attention on how this impeded his ability to advance and at certain times, how it resulted in his being "knocked off his path" toward reaching his goal.

3   How much easier it is to parent a successful Son rather than one that is having trouble.

While much of our discussion centered on parallel or isomorphic structures through verbal double *entendres* (e.g., the word "slack" in the rope/belay system and the word "slack" when he is doing well), there are other forms of parallel structures existing when creating effective interventions.

Another common example of a parallel process besides language is the actual physical structure of the activity (a kinesthetic double entendre instead of a verbal double entendre). Critical in working this family's experience was the position of the family members in appropriate roles. For example, given the family's story and structure, it was important to have the Mom belay while one of her Sons climbed the challenge course initiative. It is important to place the clients in the family structure that mirrors the family dynamics of the treatment plan. Selecting an appropriate activity and positioning clients in parallel roles to the clients' lives (e.g., selecting an activity that involves balance when working through school-social limits) are examples of the kinesthetic double entendre process.

Below is the link of the recording of this therapy session. The recording was shown at a professional development workshop sponsored by the National Association of Social Workers of Maine: https://www.youtube.com/watch?v=XmXcZO6jpcA.

Guideposts for isomorphic framing

1   Isomorphic framing requires a strong sensitivity to a client's needs, an ability to co-create meaningful experiences with clients, and an understanding of how adventure therapy experiences can provide successful resolution.
2   Isomorphic framing requires prescriptive techniques in its use. This often requires a greater breadth and depth of assessment as well as an understanding of what change will mean to the client's life if it occurs.
3   The efficacy of including metaphors in an activity requires the ability to see parallel structures. It is important to practice the use of metaphors beside using them in actual practice.
4   Presenting isomorphic frameworks requires an ability to understand the client's reality. Value the client's context and other related background issues.
5   Frame activities so they are open-ended to allow for each client to internalize personal perspectives.

5 Adventure therapy
Debriefing and frontloading

One of the key elements for adventure therapists to structure into the process is the development of clients' reflections on their participation in the adventure therapy experience. Experience alone does not typically lead to a functional change by clients unless some form of reflection accompanies it. And when in therapeutic groups, reflective facilitated discussion often helps clients uncover analogous connections and accelerate functional change processes. One common questioning process in adventure therapy is the three-question process adapted from Gestalt therapy (Boyton, 1970; Priest & Gass, 2005). These three questions are:

- WHAT? = What happened?
- SO WHAT? = So, what did you learn about changing?
- NOW WHAT? = So, how will you now integrate this change into your life?

One of the advantages of this three-question format is that it mirrors stages of CHANGES. That is, the "what" questions target client responses to the *generating* part of the model, the "so what" questions focus client responses on the *evaluation* part of the model, and the "now what" questions center client attention on the *solution* part of the model.

Debriefing: The funnel model

While the "What, So what, Now what" model offers some general guidance for therapeutic debriefing, other models integrate these concepts for greater specificity and focus for adventure therapists to center client attention on targeted therapeutic issues. One such design is the funnel model (Priest & Gass, 2005; Priest, Gass, & Gillis, 2009). This model is intended to take the broad focus of general therapeutic discussion and center it on specific client reflection, integration, and continuation. In doing this, the discussion takes on the shape of a funnel where the broad range of discussion material can be concentrated down to the essential focus for functional change. With the debriefing funnel, several forms of

DOI: 10.4324/9781032640303-5

questions, or filters, are sequentially organized to screen out irrelevant issues and formally allow critical therapeutic factors to progress.

The question process with the funnel follows a six-step sequential model

From the opening general discussion, the group and the adventure therapist focus on a discussion topic (review). After discussing this topic, the adventure therapist asks for examples of where this behavior occurred in the experience (recall/remember). Based upon these examples and occurrences, the group is asked about the impact on other group members (identify impact) and what clients learned (summation). Based on all this information, attention is focused on how the meanings/learning/changes occurring in the adventure experience pertain to the clients' lives (apply) and what clients need to do to change toward functional/healthy behaviors (commit). While it is not necessary for clients to discuss each of these filters/levels for change to occur, adventure therapists generally follow this order of progression when using this model. In following this process, adventure therapists need to assess client agreement/understanding at each filter/level before moving on to the next level. This sequential filter process is diagrammed in Figure 5.1.

As seen in this diagram, the six question filters are expansions of the three basic "what," "so what," and "now what" questions presented earlier. The "what" question covers the three reflection filters of review, remember, and identify. The "so what" question addresses the two integration filters of sum up and apply. The "now what" question centers clients' attention on the continuation filter of committing to change. Again, asking questions through these six filters sequentially is recommended as a guide for supporting the integration of change into clients' lives. An example of each filter and its purpose, with sample questions around the issue of cooperation, is shown in Figure 5.2.

From the information gathered from this model, a funnel-type system can be used to locate and refine learning from debriefings of adventure therapy experiences. Think of a radio locator passing over a series of channels back and forth, looking for the correct signal to lock onto. This is referred to as the GRABBSS model for:

- G – GOALS
- R – READINESS
- A – AFFECT
- B – BEHAVIOR
- B – BODY
- S – STAGE
- S – SETTING

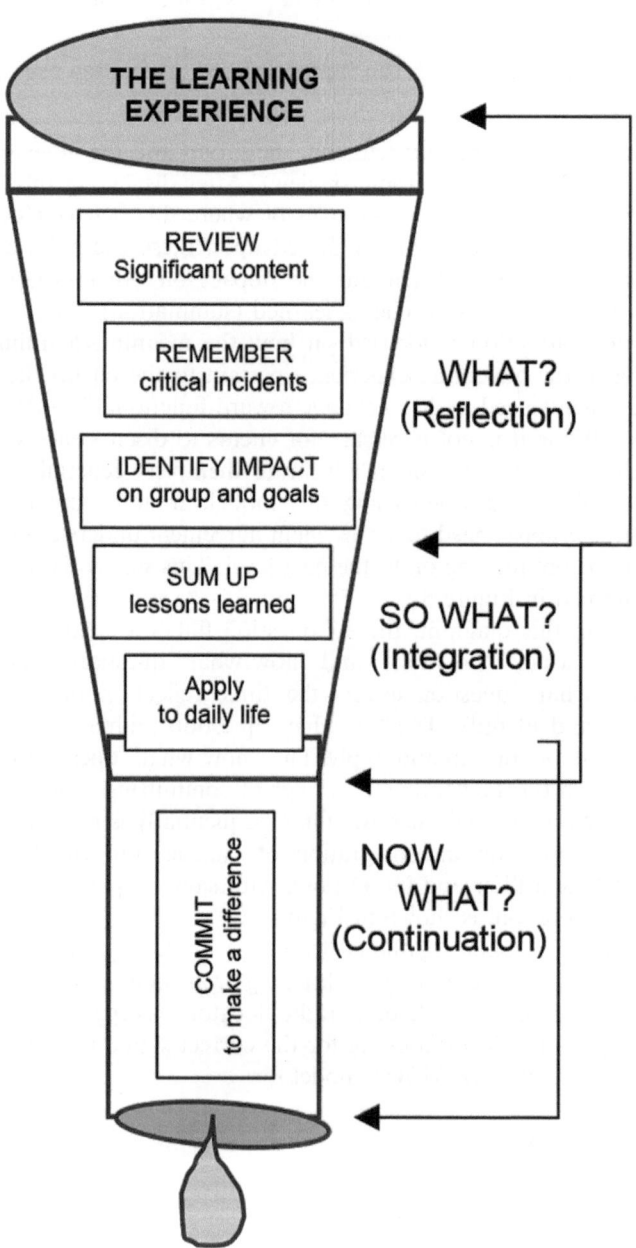

Figure 5.1 Funnel model for debriefing

Changes	Filter	Purpose	Sample Questions for Kinesthetic Metaphor
Generate	Review	Select specific topic for client discussion based on client needs.	*can you review the last activity for me?* *On a five-paint scale, hold up the number of fingers indicating how well you cooperated in the last activity.*
	Remember	Identify and agree upon elements from adventure experience pertaining to topic under discussion	*Do you remember an example of a time when the group did well in cooperating?*
Evaluate	Identify	Identify consequences relating tp emotions and changes because of client behaviors in adventure experience	*What affect did the experience have on your ability to cooperate?* *How did that emotion affect the way the group cooperated?*
	Sum Up	Summarize what clients have learned about a specific issue from an adventure experience	*Can you sum up what you gained from this experience?* *What was the moral of the story for this group?* *What are one or two key things you learned about how you cooperate?*
Seek solutions	Apply	Apply learning/change processes from adventure experiences to clients' lives	*How can you apply the way you cooperated in this experience back at you home?* *Do you see any connections rom the learning in this activity to your life back home?*
	Commit	Identity how clients will continue and commit to positive changes occuring in the adveture experience	*How can you commit to the changes in cooperation you have suggested?* *Who will help support you in your commitment to cooperate back home?*

Figure 5.2 Solution orientated facilitation in debriefing

This second form of structured reflective questioning is called solution-oriented facilitation. Research has shown solution-oriented approaches to be very effective when combined with adventure experiences, particularly with dys-functional groups (Gass & Priest, 2006; Gass & Gillis, 1995). It is important to note two critical elements of this method of processing. First, solution-oriented facilitation does *not* ignore clients' problems but seeks to address them by using different focuses than are traditionally used by many therapists. Second, solu-tion-oriented facilitation is not just "thinking positively" about situations. It seeks to address clients' issues through several key steps of questioning about clients' issues. These can include how to handle problems well, "exceptions" when problems don't occur or occur less frequently.

Frontloading adventure therapy experiences

With debriefing or funneling, the focus of dialogue or questions centers on the reaction to completed adventure experiences and narrowing down information to two or three central concepts. In reverse-like fashion, frontloading involves identifying key questions before the activity or learning experience that allow clients to identify and expand their thoughts and efforts. "Front" indicates that the facilitation occurs upfront or before the experience. "Loading" refers to the fact that the learning is loaded together, or emphasized, in combination before-hand. Frontloading centers on punctuating the key learning points in advance of the adventure experience rather than reviewing or debriefing learning afterward. Frontloading typically utilizes one or more of the following six types of ques-tions: revisiting, objectives, motivation, function, dysfunction, and prediction.

In fact, some of the most important assessment questions a therapist could ask a client would be around this concept of free framing the experience to not only learn what the clients will see as beneficial change but also frame the client's attention around what will be the center of change. Asking these questions in a story-blind way will sometimes free the mind and body to recenter attention around the therapeutic objectives. For example, the following question proactively frontloads the attention of the therapist and client to the therapeutic objective:

> *"Let me ask you a question that may help us determine what we'd like to center on in therapy before we get started. Let's think ahead to your car ride back home, and most certainly, one of you will turn to the other and ask the proverbial question you know you will be asked. Something like, 'So what did you think of that day-to-day that we centered on this therapeutic objective?' And you turn back to the questioner and respond, 'It was great! It was even better than I thought it was going to be. Because we focused on* this, *we centered on* this, *and we addressed* these *types of issues. In fact, I didn't think we would do as well as we did, but certain behaviors and springing certain questions on one another were incredibly valuable.' What must happen for you to respond in this way? What do people have to do to respond in this way? And not because you wanted me to feel good as your facilitator, but this is what you truly feel like on this ride home today after our activity."*

In fact, before you even begin therapeutic sessions or beginnings, asking the client this question in this manner could prove incredibly valuable in directing your therapeutic movement and objectives. And just like debriefing is to frontload, treatment objectives are related to proactive or framing activities. Another example of a proactive framing approach could be the following:

> *"We all had a pretty good session today and worked hard. Some of us sweated a lot, cried some, and hopefully didn't bleed much, but when we get home, you know you're going to have to do a few things, one of which is take a shower* (this introduction usually solicits some laughter and smiles). *But as you shower, you know the dirt will go down the proverbial drain. But there are some things that you want to prevent from going down the drain. These are things you want to keep, remember, learn from, and center your attention and objectives on. What are the things you want to ensure don't go down the drain later today and you want to carry with you as great learnings from each other today?"*

The excitement of adventure activities can help a group focus intensely on completing a task, distracting it from the changes it is there to accomplish. These revisiting questions remind group members of the behaviors they pledged to perform after the last activity. Just before the new activity begins and after you have explained the task, you can pose a single question: *"One more thing. What were the commitments the group made last time?"* This brief question brings the previous answers to the "do things differently next time" question to the front of their clients' minds so they are likely to act on their revisited affirmations during the activity.

Besides a revisiting question, you can ask the types of frontloading questions in any combination or alone. Revisiting questions reminds the group of the behaviors they pledged to follow after the last activity. Motivation questions focus on the "Why" of an activity. This may be important on how this learning relates to daily life. Objective questions ask about the goals of the activity and what will be gained from the experience. Functional questions are those that identify and develop how the group may optimize their strengths and resources. Dysfunctional questions ask what behaviors will hinder success and how the group can avoid or overcome them. Prediction questions ask clients to imagine what is going to happen. These six question types for frontloading are like the six questions posed as filters in the funneling model. The difference between frontloading and funneling questions is when they are asked. Frontloading questions come before the experience. Funneling questions come after the experience.

The six question types can be illustrated in the wall activity. This activity includes a 12 to 14-foot (three to four-meter) structure with a ledge on the back side. The group is challenged to pass members up the front and over the top. Getting the first person up is a challenging aspect of getting over the wall. Generally, the crux of the problem is getting the

Types of frontloading	Examples of frontloading
Revisiting	In the last activity we ended up by saying there were certain things that were key for you to be successful. Does anyone remember what those things were, and can you think of how to use them?
Motivation	What would energize you to be successful with this activity?
Objectives	What are the objectives of this task?
Function	What will you be doing that shows that you are being successful? What strengths will you use to be successful?
Dysfunction	What things do you want to avoid? How will you address challenges?
Evidence	If you are successful, what will you have said, what would you have done, what would you have thought, how would you have been thinking, and what would you have accomplished?

Figure 5.3 Types of frontloading

last person over the wall with one remaining below to lift them. In a typical discussion before the activity, you've introduced the problem by mentioning to the group the goal of getting everyone over the wall. You then review the safety procedures (e.g., not holding on to the side edges, no more than two people on the ledge at a time, not holding people upside down).

Below are six examples of frontloading and how it is used effectively in adventure experiences (Figure 5.3).

The structural process fostering the development of reflection possesses several common elements. These elements include: (1) fostering reflective discussions by asking questions as a facilitator, (2) creating group structures for reflective discussions that foster instructive dialogue, (3) using appropriate discussion guidelines to foster constructive dialogue for reflection, (4) following the "do's and don'ts" of adventure therapy reflective questioning, (5) creating an appropriate therapeutic atmosphere for reflective discussions, and (6) managing client information for reflective discussions.

6 Gift giving

Imagine it's your friend's birthday and you are at their party. The time has come in the celebration process to give birthday gifts. As we have all observed in the past there can be a variety of responses to this process. What response occurs from your client depends as much on the gift itself as well as how the gift is given. Perhaps you have seen some of these situations.

1 Despite your best intentions, your gift just didn't seem to be something they liked, wanted, or needed.
2 As the gift is opened up your friend finds the gift of value, but it's just not quite right (e.g., the gift is the wrong size). So, you say, "The gift receipt is in the box if you want to return it" to try and salvage the situation.
3 The gift you gave is greatly appreciated, but the way you gave it was awkward. Much of the meaning for this gift was lost because of how it is presented.
4 Your friend is excited about opening the gift because of the joke you said as you gave it and when it is opened everyone can tell it is perfect. In a heartfelt way your friend says "How did you know? This is exactly what I wanted! It is perfect! Thanks so much!"

These scenarios are similar to how a metaphor is presented to a client. Zeig (1992, 1994) and Itin (2001) have applied gift giving concepts (e.g., gift wrapping, tailoring, processing) in their development of the Ericksonian Diamond. Both the content (i.e., what the gift is) and story (i.e., how it is presented) of the metaphor and the process or adventure activity are key for how engaged the client is to the parallel structure, kinesthetic elements, and the client's treatment goals.

The interaction between these two variables can be seen in Figure 6.1 with the gift being a "rock." In quadrant #1, the lower left-hand corner of the figure occurs when the presenter has missed on both the value of the gift and its presentation. In quadrant #2, the delivery is meaningful, but the value of the gift leaves a lot to be desired. In quadrant #3, the value of

DOI: 10.4324/9781032640303-6

Rock giving activity	Poor or inappropriate delivery	Great or meaningful delivery
Great content or value	#3 "This is really beautiful and I really like it, but did you have to give me lingerie in front of all these people?"	#4 The gift giver, "I remembered what you told me last month." The receiver, "This is exactly what I wanted! I can't believe you could find it!"
Poor content or value	#1 "Oh, my…. hmm… I can't believe you gave me this. I thought you knew about my allergy. Maybe next time just ask me so everyone doesn't have a laugh."	#2 "Gee, this is really nice, but I think I need a different size. I guess I can return it and get something else."

Figure 6.1 Content (product) and delivery (process) for adventure experiences in general

the gift is high, but the delivery undermines the gift. It is only in quadrant #4, where both the value of the gift and a meaningful delivery combine to represent a comprehensive message.

The gift of a rock: Practicing the delivery of kinesthetic metaphor content and meaning

One way of developing rich content and meaning in the substance and delivery of kinesthetic metaphors is to practice. One way of learning how to create transderivational searches is to practice "gift giving." This exercise asks therapists to think of a person they would like to acknowledge with a message written on a small rock or stone (e.g., "You show compassion"). In many ways the introduction to this practice exercise is parallel/similar to the process of inducing transderivational search.

Before clients select their rocks, I provide them with examples of what they might want to do as well as what they might want to avoid. For example, I start the exercise by simply walking up and placing a rock in a volunteer's hand. Without explanation, they blankly look at me and say: "What's this for?" (see quadrant #1 in Figure 6.2). I then take the rock back and begin to share attributes that I appreciate and value about this person (e.g., "You are a responsible person who is dedicated in helping

Rock giving activity	Bad or inappropriate delivery	Great or meaningful delivery
Great content or value	#3 "I like the $500 that rock would bring me, but if I try and catch it the way you are going to throw it is really going to hurt!"	#4 "The things you said about me leave me speechless. There is a place on my mantle that I will keep this rock forever."
Poor content or value	#1 "What's this rock for? Why did you give it to me?"	#2 "It really was kind of you to say all of that about me, but I don't get why you gave me a rock?"

Figure 6.2 Rock giving for content (product) and delivery (process)

young people..."). Then I walk up and hand them the rock, and while they are thankful for my comments, they still are left wondering "Why did he give me this rock?" (See quadrant #2 in Figure 6.2).

I then take a few steps back so there is about 10 meters between myself and the "volunteer." I explain that this rock is quite expensive, worth about $500 at a local rock store. I start to mimic some warm-up throwing gestures like a baseball pitcher would do to a catcher, making it clear that my intention is to throw the rock as fast as I can. Not only does the volunteer start to grimace and move out of the way, anyone else behind this person also begins to duck their heads. In many ways this interaction mirrors the action of recipients in quadrant #3. Of course, what I am really after is giving a meaningful delivery with a metaphorical personalization of the rock to the receiver (see quadrant #4 in Figure 6.2). At this time, I show the assortment of rocks that are available for participants to select, letting them know there is a rock that will fit every person. Markers can be used to write personal inscriptions or draw meaningful designs: tailoring the rock specifically to the individual.

Case study of gift giving #1 – Leaving rocks behind: Post-traumatic stress disorder with combat soldiers serving in Afghanistan

I was contacted by a colleague serving as a Captain in the US Army in Afghanistan. His base commander, clinical psychologists, and he were concerned that the "recovery" process for their soldiers in the next few months didn't seem effective. They asked for assistance in designing an adventure therapy-based program that could help enrich this process. With their guidance we designed an 8–12-week program involving returning soldiers in appropriate and structured adventure experiences (e.g., climbing, paddling, backpacking, community picnics, and service projects) (see Gass, Gillis, & Russell, 2020).

One of the activities pivotal for several soldiers, addressed the "weight" of the post-traumatic stress they continued to face while in combat. Soldiers spoke freely about certain elements they would like to "leave behind" when they complete their deployment and return home.

To address this, we invited soldiers to participate in an experience that identified the level of "weight/stress" from combat and to consider steps in being able to leave these experiences behind. At the beginning of the week, we asked each soldier to find a rock that represented the amount of "weight" that they were carrying in their backpack. Almost every soldier selected a rock and placed it in their backpack. Right before we were ready to begin the hike up the mountain, soldiers were informed they could stop the group at any time to talk about their rock (e.g., what it meant, what they wanted to do with it).

Two hours into the hike one of the soldiers asked the group to stop because he wanted to discuss his rock. He pulled it out of his backpack and said that it represented the guilt he was experiencing because he felt that the death of one of the soldiers in the company was his fault. He wanted to let everyone know about his pain and guilt around their fellow soldier's death and to ask for forgiveness.

After a slight pause, one of his closest comrades gently spoke from his heart stating it wasn't his fault. He continued to say that it wasn't anyone's fault in the company. He just had bad luck and was in the wrong place at the wrong time. The swell of comments from other soldiers firmly agreed the soldier who spoke out, stating that even if it was his fault, all was forgiven and the bond between soldiers grew even further in perspective. Some of the soldiers in the company encouraged him to leave the rock behind, or at the very least take a lighter rock instead. With a new rock in his pack, the soldier asked for forgiveness and continued down the trail with an "uplifted" pack.

Case study of gift giving #2 – Leaving rocks behind: Making decisions to move from powerlessness to control

This activity was developed during a consultation with a colleague about a client she was working with who was particularly "stuck." This adolescent woman had a history of abandonment and was a victim of verbal and physical abuse. The resulting issues included guilt, feelings of worthlessness, and an inability to let go and move on.

The goal of this kinesthetic metaphor was to: (1) create a parallel situation where the physical weight of rocks would serve as a metaphor for her guilt that was "weighing her down" on a daily basis; (2) emphasize her ability to determine and choose daily goals associated with cognition, affect, and behaviors; and (3) help her develop a sense of choice in the way she lived.

The activity consisted of going for a walk with the client. To set up the activity, the therapist gathered a group of rocks that were of a manageable weight challenge, yet uncomfortable to carry. The client was asked to select and carry a rock in a backpack that represented the things in her life that were weighing her down.

Debriefing this activity focused on her decision to not put on the backpack. We discussed feelings of what it would be like to wear it and what it would be like to not wear it. These discussions led to the insight of having to make choices in her life. Through this activity, the client was able to take ownership over her choices.

7 Two case studies

Substance use relapse prevention

This chapter of the book focuses on presenting two case studies on the therapeutic issue of adolescent substance abuse relapse prevention. Each case study uses one or more experiential techniques to construct a strong intervention to address this therapeutic issue.

Effective treatments of behavioral healthcare issues with adolescents have never been as needed as they are today. Seven out of 10 adolescents in the United States currently identify anxiety or depression as a personal issue, with 75% of high school students expressing boredom, anger, sadness, fear, or distress while in school (Bouchrika, 2023). The most diagnosed mental disorders in children ages 3–17 years, from 2016–2019, were attention deficit hyperactivity disorder (9.8%), anxiety (9.4%), behavioral problems (8.9%), and depression (4.4%) (CDC, 2023). From 2007 to 2018, suicide rates among youth ages 10–24 in the United States increased by 57%, with 6,600 deaths by suicide among the 10–24 age group in 2020 (Curtin, 2020). And of the 7.7 million children with treatable mental health disorders, 50% did not receive adequate treatment in 2016 (Child Focus, 2022). Despite the best efforts to address these issues, these devastating trends continue unabated.

Figures outside of the United States are not much different. Almost one in every seven adolescents experience mental health difficulties, and one adolescent loses their life every 11 minutes to suicide. Anxiety and depression in youth, ages 10–19, comprise 40% of all adolescents experiencing mental health issues (UNICEF, 2022).

When adolescents begin to experience therapeutic issues of depression (e.g., DSM-5 296.20–36, ICD-10 code F-32.0–33.3), anxiety (e.g., DSM-5 300.02 [F41.1], DSM 309.24 [F43, 22]), suicidal ideation (ICD-10-R45.851) or other therapeutic issues, their families typically turn first to standard treatment programs (e.g., office therapies, outpatient treatment) using standardized therapy practices (e.g., cognitive behavioral therapies). When these practices fail to help the client or the client's issues become overly acute, families often turn to residential treatment care (e.g., congregate care). In the last 5 years, there has been a 25% decline in private treatment (NATSAP, 2022).

DOI: 10.4324/9781032640303-7

Case study #1 - Putting it all together: Intersecting adventure therapy models for even greater change

Adventure therapy tends to be most effective when all three phases of facilitation (i.e., assessment, intervention, debriefing) are brought together. One of the most influential adventure therapy experiences, especially with substance abusers, is the Maze initiative. First developed in 1988 at the Eagleville Hospital in Eagleville, Pennsylvania, this therapeutic experience was initially created for adults with substance use issues. When done correctly, it typically resolves at least two key elements in the treatment of substance users. However, when used incorrectly, clients often feel "deceived, outraged, humiliated, and shamed for not getting the right answer" (Porter, 1989, p. 88).

This therapeutic experience is best used with groups that center on the pre-contemplative stage of development in the theoretical change model. For example, with clients in the pre-contemplative state, centering attention on specific areas of substance abuse relapse may not be accepted by clients.

One treatment model that synergistically intersects with the Maze experience is the Transtheoretical Model of Change (e.g., states of precontemplation, action, relapse). Presented in this manner, the treatment emphasizes: 1) the ability of substance abusers to ask for help and 2) their ability to set appropriate boundaries around issues concerning their recovery and maintaining abstinence. In Figure 7.1 you can see how the client's readiness to change greatly effects how you facilitate an activity. For example, clients centered in the precontemplation belief stage shouldn't be expected to see how the maze is connected to their substance use. Instead, they should be exposed to a belief system that offers a range of outcomes in the activity like the presence of outcomes in their current life. So, focusing of more applicable and pertinent objectives will focus more effectively on treatment goals.

Another critical area, particularly in systemic thinking, is the sacrifice of some family members for others. For example, with some families there are individuals who will maintain substance use patterns for the benefit of staying connected to others in the family. For us at Eagleville Hospital, this occurred with families where the woman was at the center of the family system and would sacrifice herself for other family members.

The set-up for this initiative is the same as the Maze initiative except for how an exit from the maze is created. Individuals are blindfolded, introduced to the initiative by a metaphorical description of the experience, and led by the instructors to various points in the maze. The participants have yet to see the maze area prior to the activity, and the usual precautions for safety are taken (e.g., no ducking under the ropes, making sure the area is clear of debris and branches, one hand holds onto the rope and the other hand is up in front like a bumper should someone be close to you).

The following is a sample presentation of the metaphor experience:

Transtheortical Model of Change	Likely thoughts or behaviors of client	Therapist's facilitation focus
Precontemplation	Unaware of behavior problems or negative consequences. Underestimates benefits of change. No intention of change.	Stay group-centered, introduce the concept that the activity's outcome may be one of multiple possibilities. Be prepared for possible tension or ambivalence.
Contemplation	Intends to start healthy behavior Recognizes behavior may be problematic. Getting ready to consider change.	Compare outcomes, examine how change benefits client.
Preparation	Ready to take action. Takes small steps toward behavioral change.	Continue to support client's behavioral change. Help client recognize the benefits of their new behaviors.
Action	Behavioral changes have been made. Intenda to keep on this path.	Identify what needs to be continued to support behavioral changes. Highlight the benefits of choosing healthier behaviors.
Maintenance	Sustains behavioral change for 6 months or more. Intends to continue with behavioral change.	Acknowledge client's success with behavioral changes. Recognize potential triggers that could evoke relapse.
Termination	Client states no desire to return to unhealthy behaviors. Confident that change has solified into their life.	Reinforce their successes and recognize their strategies to maintain healthy behaviors.

Figure 7.1 Transtheoretical model of change

"*The next activity is called the Path to Recovery. It's called that because several of the obstacles you'll encounter in this experience are very similar to obstacles many of you are currently encountering in your addictions. Our addictions often blind us on our path to a substance-free lifestyle, and we often fail because we don't remember to live by the principles that allow us to free ourselves from abusive substances. We will place you on the road to recovery by putting your hand onto a rope. This rope will lead you along a path of interminable length. Along your journey to recovery, you will meet various other people going in different directions. Some of these people will be in a great hurry, showing a lot of confidence. Others will be tentative, moving cautiously. Some will seem to know the right direction, whereas others will seem lost. Don't let go of the rope! Because if you do, you will lose the path, and we will ask you to sit down until the initiative ends.*

The goal of your journey is to reach the exit of this maze. You'll know that you are at the exit because when you reach the exit, I will tap you on the shoulder and ask you to make an important choice. The choice will be either: 1) step out of the maze (if you decide to step out, I'll ask you to remove your blindfold and sit quietly in the abstinence area until this initiative is over); or 2) you can choose to go back to the maze to help others. If you choose to go back into the maze, you run the risk that this exit may be shut when you return.

If at any time during this activity you would like to receive help, all you need to do is ask for it, and guidance will be provided. Otherwise, we would like everyone to avoid speaking throughout this initiative until it's completed.

Remember the rules of this initiative:
Follow the safety rules.
Speak only if you would like some help.
I will be waiting for you at the exit of the maze to ask you if you want to go back in.

After approximately 30 minutes, I will ask those still in the maze to remove their blindfolds for a small break."

Participants are distributed throughout the maze and instructed not to move until the "go ahead" is given. When everyone has been placed in the maze, participants are informed that they can begin to try and find an exit. In this initiative, however, all exits remain closed until at least one person asks for "help." Doing so opens the exits, and the person asking for help is directed toward the open exit.

When participants arrive at an exit, they are quietly asked to make their decision. Instructors should do this without revealing the location of the exit to other participants. If the participants choose to step out, they are asked to quietly remove their blindfolds and step aside to observe others in the maze. It is important for these participants not to wander off but to remain and be silent observers of the process. If the participants choose to go back into the maze, this exit closes, and the instructor should proceed. Exits may open and close quite often if participants continually make this choice. If participants become grouped near the exit, allow each person to make their decision before adhering to the "exit rotation" rule.

Some participants may still be in the maze after the 30-minute limit, usually because they keep going back into the maze to rescue one another, even though each may have found an exit at least once. It's a judgment call whether to keep permitting people to continually go back into the maze after 30 minutes. Still, I usually stop the initiative at 30 minutes if everyone has made it to an exit at least once to make their decision. At this point, I ask participants in the maze to quietly remove their blindfolds and come and join the rest of the group in a circle.

As for debriefing, different issues come up with each group, but I usually begin the initiative by asking people to relate their experience in the initiative to their experience in trying to reach or maintain sobriety. A variety of issues come up, but the primary ones focused on are (1) how asking for help assisted people in this initiative, (2) people's choices at the exits, and (3) what "failing to hold on" to the rope represented. As stated earlier, if using a model like the transtheoretical one discussed above, the focus of the discussion while debriefing is often determined by the clients' stage of change at that stage.

In the discussion, I inform people that exits weren't opened until someone asked for help and describe how asking for help directed this person to an exit. I also asked this person to elaborate on why they asked for help and what it felt like to receive assistance. The whole point of including this dynamic and the initiative is to link the parallel experiences together.

The "choice" decision is meant to metaphor a critical boundary issue for substance abusers. These clients must place their recovery process first in any decision. To step out of the maze represents a healthy personal decision. To choose to go back in represents a dangerous decision, one where they may never achieve an exit to abstinence again.

Sometimes, people (e.g., adolescents) state that they stayed in the maze because "stepping out" would be "boring." This is key to discuss since abstinence may seem less exciting than "being in the game." However, this game has tragic consequences for users, which is important to discuss.

Some other important metaphors include:

- To "let go" of the rope is to lose a chance to achieve abstinence
- The feelings of people observing others "lost" in the maze of abusive substances
- Implementing the metaphorical techniques participants used to "find an exit" to abstinence
- Interaction with others searching for abstinence in the maze
- The inability to communicate while searching for abstinence
- The role of the hospitals/treatment centers in "placing" clients on the road to abstinence, and the role of the client to follow the path and make choices
- Many more occur; don't stay limited to these!

Case study #2 - The pinning ceremony

Key to the experiential learning cycle is the reflection period following the learning experience. Probably some of the most powerful of these are graduation and other ceremonial closure experiences. Outward bound is one of the longest running programs that uses pins to symbolize the successful completion of an Outward Bound course. The granting of these pins highlights the processes of the pinning ceremony.

Another such use of pinning as a key element and common ritual of the substance abuse community is the granting of pins or a pinning ceremony to indicate the number of days of abstinence for drug users. "An AA medallion is a symbolic token that Alcoholics Anonymous members receive to mark the passage of specific amounts of time since they consumed alcohol. The practice dates to 1942 when a man named Doherty S. started an AA gathering in Indianapolis. (Anonymity is the foundation of AA so no last names are shared.)" (AA, p. 2).

The idea of the pinning ritual in adventure therapy is to not take away from the strength of the Outward Bound or AA model, but to utilize the strengths and traditions of these two influential programs. Prior to the experience, the therapist purchases/gathers symbolic pins for the participants. With participants sitting in the circle, the therapist facilitates a general overview and summary of the clients' experience. The concepts and ideas shared at this time generally focus on learning and reflecting on the experiences shared together and pass with thoughts on how this will continue to stay strong once everyone goes their separate ways. Toward the end of this dialogue, the therapist takes some time to spread out the pins in front of everyone and allows them to examine them. After people view the pins, they are asked to consider who should receive such a pin and why. Participants are invited to present a pin to a person as a symbol of their being, effort, and accomplishments in the AA experience. After starting the presentation, other group members may add additional comments as gifts to the person who received the pin. If the recipient has any clarification questions on the comments they are hearing, they are encouraged to respond. Other than these comments participants usually focus on listening to what is being given to them in terms of verbal gifts. If the pins are all the same, comments seem more unified and similar. If they are different, comments are more symbolic around the characteristics shared by the pin. Given this, identical pins seem to make more sense for the group who doesn't know each other well, different pins for groups who do. This is why the AA pin seems to work well. Therapists are sometimes included in their pinning ceremony when appropriate. Some of the most common reflective exercises that can be combined with the pins are closure experiences. Additional reflective exercises can be combined with the pinning exercise.

Following the pinning, a therapist might include a metaphorical "leaving it behind" experience. This additional experience could include 20–30 minutes of a "solo" experience. Framing up this exercise works best if therapists initiate, early in treatment, the concept of making necessary positive changes. The "glue" that allows the exercise to "stick" is provided by the continuity built into the program by its leaders.

Sample presentation at the edge of a stream

> *"Take 10–15 minutes now while you sit at the water's edge to reflect on the decisions and the challenges you have thought about taking home with you from your session. As the water passes by you on its steady course, consider what new things you have learned about yourself: How your life has changed? What will it be like to return to your life with newfound strength?"*
>
> (Long pause)
>
> *"See the water as a body on a similar path. Upstream, the water is different than it is in front of you and still different downstream from where you now sit. Along its path, it supports different animal and plant life, and it changes speed and direction along the way. The river continues to adapt and flow despite all the things thrown into it.*
>
> *Just as the river fluctuates with the environment, so can you. As part of altering your own course, you will soon throw your chosen old behavior/decisions away and create a new set of behavior/decisions for yourself. When you are ready, throw that bundle into the water of the past and see yourself beginning anew, ready to navigate uncharted waters."*

Debriefing

I think the best way to leave this activity is to walk away from it in silence without debriefing, perhaps coming back to a circle where food or drink is waiting. This way, the very intimate nature of the personal decisions can be honored. Younger people may need more assistance directing their reflection time.

8 Working with clients who present difficulties

Most of the techniques outlined in this book can successfully be utilized without significant difficulty. This is usually the case when clients are fully involved in adventure experiences. However, despite the best intentions by an adventure therapist, things do not always proceed as planned. When clients appear to be experiencing challenges, adventure therapists need to provide the necessary adjustments to enhance change opportunities.

One critical element for working with clients experiencing challenges is to understand their behavior is not usually directed at you but at the emotions, thoughts, and actions they are facing. Remaining neutral, supportive, objective, and impartial in resolving difficult issues can often be a major source of assistance for clients when they need you the most.

Clients involved in dysfunctional situations

Dysfunctional behaviors occur when clients find themselves unable to produce healthy actions and behaviors (Gass, Gillis, & Russell, 2020). Clients generally don't present these behaviors because of potential consequences (e.g., the loss in social status, interacting with an authority figure). Note that dysfunctional client behaviors are not always consequential (e.g., not getting caught when drinking underage, having the resources available to avoid incarceration). Therapists should try to view dysfunctional behaviors as potential "solutions" that can be constructed into more appropriate or effective "paths." While this perspective may be difficult, adventure therapists who take such a "stance" or perspective can provide a much richer resource for healthy change with clients, especially ones who are disempowered.

There are three key prerequisites that should be revisited before addressing dysfunctional behaviors. The first is to build a therapeutic relationship that includes such things as avoiding judgement, listening with intention to what is being said and the feelings behind the words, and being present to the client's experiences. The second prerequisite is having a clear awareness and agreement on why certain dynamics have placed them in dysfunctional situations. And the third is the understanding of why they are in therapy with therapeutic goals.

DOI: 10.4324/9781032640303-8

Identifying and addressing dysfunctional behaviors

Successful therapy involves a strong understanding of the therapeutic process. However, there are times when clients and therapists may disagree with parts of the therapeutic process resulting in dysfunctional behaviors. These dysfunctional behaviors can present themselves as different feelings, behaviors, or belief systems. Four of these dysfunctional behaviors include: disagreeing, resistance, denying, and being apathetic.

Disagreeing clients understand the purpose of the therapeutic activity (e.g., walking a maze), but disagree on why or how they will be involved (e.g., don't want to wear a blindfold). To resolve this issue the therapist needs to have an honest and open relationship to reach a common ground. Facilitating the group to a position where they listen to one another and share different ideas are important functional models for healthy behaviors. Once all positions are presented, adventure therapists seek to affiliate and empathize with clients for discussion. Again, disagreement can be a highly positive benefit of client work. However, if cohesiveness leads to unhealthy or unproductive decisions, combined with a lack of awareness of issues, then adventure therapists should examine resistance as a source of the problematic behavior.

Resistant clients state they don't want to participate in the therapeutic activity regardless of how much additional information or negotiation is offered. Clients understand their therapeutic work, but resistance is shown by their reduction in the quantity, content, style, and logistics of their therapeutic process (Otani, 1989). These four characteristics are enhanced through adventure therapy because the activities are often kinesthetic, challenging, adventurous, involve group work, occur in nature, and use metaphoric processes. One way to address client resistance is by utilizing the "confusion technique" (Otani, 1989). Here, using a questioning process, the adventure therapist asks the clients to help the therapist understand the clients' value behind such a resistant position. The following are a couple of questions that could be asked by an adventure therapist to address client resistance through the confusion technique:

> *"...you know, I have done this adventure experience with probably over 100 groups before today. And I have never seen a group respond to the presenting problem like your group did today. It would be interesting to hear from the group why they responded like they did..."*

After some explanation from clients to this response, if the adventure therapist still believes clients are resistant to presenting valid responses, the therapist can continue with this confusion technique with questions like the following:

"I don't think I am truly understanding what you are trying to say. Is there another way you can explain your reasoning to me?"

The "confusion technique" aims to have clients project ever-increasing clarifying responses to the reasoning behind their behaviors. When this occurs the client's resistant behavior tends to lose its strength and reason for existence. If a client's resistance is still present, adventure therapists can work with the client to see if there is a part of the activity that they can connect with in a solution-orientated manner.

When clients are in denial, they appear to be in a state of opposition to therapy. The main construction of denial behavior is that clients won't accept the changes offered to them because they deny having a problem (Sutton, 2021). Many of these individuals are in Prochaska and Velicer's (1997) pre-contemplative stage of change, where they avoid the topic, don't believe they have a problem, make excuses or rationalizations, and often blame others for their problem.

Adventure therapy provides some distinct advantages for the therapeutic process. One of these is the use of natural consequences to punctuate therapeutic change (e.g., if a client doesn't wear a jacket, they will get cold). As clients continue to encounter these "natural" consequences, it becomes increasingly difficult to deny the obvious outcomes of their maladaptive behavior. As their dysfunctional behavior becomes more apparent, they begin to see the need to take responsibility and change their behavior. The logical connection between their actions and consequences becomes more difficult to deny.

As a dysfunctional behavior, apathy describes those clients who don't care to change regardless of a particular benefit. In all other types of difficult behavior, clients' motivation is available to some extent, but misguided. The main issue with apathetic clients is that they possess little motivation to change, and they are often in a state of learned helplessness. Adventure therapists should make sure their initial prerequisites (i.e., strong therapeutic relationship, clear reason for therapy, achievable goals) are well visited and understood. Once this occurs, the vigorous learning environment of an adventure experience, combined with a solution-oriented approach, promotes a treatment advantage possessed by adventure therapy over other forms of therapy.

One such technique that supports the use of an "antidote" to dysfunctional behaviors is the use of "proactive reframing" (a form of the miracle question). This therapeutic process takes advantage of clients' reflecting on their behavior even before it begins. The conversation by the therapist could go something like this:

THERAPIST: "One of the questions you will probably be asked by a close friend/partner is, *'How was that adventure thing you did yesterday? What happened? Did it help you?'*

"So, if I (therapist) were that friend/partner, what would you say to me that would explain what must happen for you to say that it was great, successful, powerful, etc.?" (i.e., proactive reframing using a form the miracle question.)

When the therapist asks this hypothetical question, they are attempting to create a solution-focused, pre-experience front-load for the client.

Two key elements of this therapeutic technique provide rich sources of information that can prove valuable in resolving dysfunctional behaviors and meeting therapeutic goals. First, the technique gives the client some ideas and directions about where the therapeutic process may take them in their future adventure therapy experience. Second, it tells the therapist what the client is expecting to happen and what would make the session successful. Another advantage in using this technique is that it bypasses client resistance because you are discussing a therapeutic experience that has not yet occurred. Figure 8.1 shows a summary of the four types of problematic behaviors, their basic characteristics, and some action strategies employed by an adventure therapist:

Other forms of difficult behavior (e.g., silent, controlling) may also exist with various clients. Some of these can include clients who are silent, possess control issues, have high levels of anxiety, are angry, hostile, or inactive. Each of these issues has its own elements that need to be addressed. Some suggestions are offered here to work with these clients, but as with all clients, the individual characteristics of their presenting problem also need to be considered.

Silent clients

There may be a variety of reasons why some clients do not speak. One of the first things adventure therapists should try to do with such clients is find out the reason for their silence. Reasons could include cultural expectations, fear, shame, reluctance, poor self-value, etc. A "good first step" in such situations is to dialogue individually with the client and find out the best way to proceed with them. If their silence is related to fear/retribution, this must be dealt with before a person can freely speak. Think about the following statement and find out if it is true in your clients' belief systems:

"If you can't say no without fear, your yes responses don't count."

What this statement means is that if clients are in situations where the conditions of their responses are tempered or negatively affected by consequences from someone else, all their responses are going to be prejudiced by this situation. Obviously, addressing these situations before continuing further therapy is very important for the growth and safety of the client.

Also know there are different ways to contribute to group or individual therapy other than speaking. Some of them include nonverbal responses

Dysfunctional Behavior	Client's Belief Structure	Therapist's Response Strategies
Disagreeing	"I understand the activity, but I want to XXX instead."	Negotiate a plan with consideration of client's best interests.
Resisting	"I understand the activity, but I'm not doing it."	Show true confusion and utilize paradoxical methods.
Denying	"I get the activity, I don't care if I really can do it, I still don't want to do it."	Be sincere, validate feelings, and ask how they may see themselves contribute to the activity? Ask what part of the activity they can connect with?
Apathetic	"There's nothing you can do that will change my mind. I'm don't want to be here."	Before the adventure experience use proactive reframing. Follow trauma informed care practices. Offer options of being in the presence of the activity (e.g., serve as a "professional observer")

Figure 8.1 Four types of problematic behaviors and their resolution

(thumbs up or thumbs down, scaling with fingers from one to ten), writing, reflection, smaller groups settings (solo, partner, triads), closed or choice questions versus open-ended questions, etc. Adventure therapists should seek the medium of communication that works best for their client.

Controlling client

Perhaps the opposite of a silent client is a controlling client who monopolizes a large degree of the therapeutic experience. This individual will often try and control the group through discussion, behavior, or other actions. In many ways, their controlling efforts serve the same function as the silence in other clients: to try and control the direction of therapy and what is discussed, and more importantly what is prevented from being discussed, in the therapeutic experience.

Your response to this type of client as an adventure therapist is much the same as with a silent client. First is to make your client aware of their controlling behavior, simply by asking if they can "share the airtime" with others in the group or by participating in activities that provide evidence of their behavior obvious to them. Priest, Gass, and Gillis (2009) provide the following suggested facilitation activities to do this:

- Introduce a "talking object" into group discussions. This is a technique where an object (e.g., a soft Nerf ball) is held by the person speaking. If you wish to speak, you must raise your hand and obtain the "talking object" before you can speak. No one can speak without first obtaining the talking object.
- Pass out three "strike anywhere" matches to each group member. If an individual wishes to speak, they start speaking and light one of their three matches. They may speak if their match continues to burn. Once it is out, and they have run out of time, they must stop talking. Once all your three matches are used up, you must wait until everyone else in the group has used up their matches before you can speak again.
- Create a literal "sociogram" with a ball of yarn. As one person speaks the ball of yarn is tossed to them. This person holds on to the ball of yarn until they are done speaking. The yarn ball is tossed to the next person who wishes to speak. This process creates a literal diagram of who speaks and how often.
- Have an external group of people observe the group process for a predetermined period and report back to the group their observations, including who speaks and how often.

These forms of process activities provide substantial feedback for the group to consider, as well as the person who may be having issues with controlling behavior. Such activities may provide enough information for the person to address their controlling behavior issues without further intervention.

Anxious client

Sometimes adventure experiences create high levels of anxiety for clients. Certainly, there are several adventure experiences that *should* create anxiety for the uninitiated participant! If the fears are related to the adventure experiences, adventure therapists can work to alleviate these fears by having clients identify them and address the reality or substance behind the fear. Again, as with many adventure therapy facilitation techniques, there are experiential methods to conduct processing. One such experiential method addressing anxiety is the "Fear in a hat" processing technique (Bell & Williams, 2006). With this experiential activity, clients gather in a circle and are directed to write down their greatest fears about the adventure therapy experience. Responses are placed in a hat and shaken to protect anonymity of client responses (i.e., no one knows which response is from which individual in the group). The group members then pull responses out of the hat one at a time and read them aloud to the group. The group discusses and analyzes the substance and reality of the fear written on the paper. The beneficial aspect of this facilitation technique is that not only does it address fears based on the adventure experiences, but it also brings to light fears concerning group issues and change processes. The resulting facilitated discussion can provide great benefits for addressing anxious client issues.

9 Adventure therapy

Transfer and research

I was driving down a local highway a while ago when I noticed the local phone company conducting training on 12–15 telephone poles with new employees whose job it was to fix telephone lines on these poles. I smiled as I thought about how students at our university were just ten miles down the road climbing 12–15 telephone poles at our challenge course with quite different objectives in mind than the phone company. One of the reasons for my smile was the thought of: "What a wonderful example of specific transfer with these line workers!" Here were new workers climbing poles to transfer these skill sets, habits, and learning associations necessary for these individuals to use these techniques in their future successfully.

When thinking of transfer, it is important to remember that transfer is a process and not an outcome. The mechanisms of transfer serve as vehicles to reach the intended outcomes of a particular participant group. And as a process, it needs to be adapted to everyone's needs. Some professionals are also confused about the difference between nonspecific transfer and metaphor transfer. Nonspecific transfer is where *specific processes* are used to connect prior learning to future learning. Metaphoric transfer is where *analogous processes* connect prior learning to future learning.

Is transferring important in adventure experiences? It depends on why you are there!

Why don't you stay in the wilderness? Because that isn't where it's at; it's back in the city, back in downtown St. Louis, back in Los Angeles. The final test is whether your experience of the sacred in nature enables you to cope more effectively with the problems of man. If it does not enable you to cope more effectively with the problems – and sometimes it doesn't, sometimes it just sucks you right out into the wilderness and you stay there the rest of your life – then when that happens, by my scale of value it's failed. You go to nature for an experience of the sacred; and I point out to you that it is not the only place that one can go, but in Outward Bound and in my own experience, it's the one that tends to be emphasized. You go there to re-establish your contact with the core of things, where it's really at, to enable you to come back into the world of man and

DOI: 10.4324/9781032640303-9

operate more effectively. So I finish with the principle: Seek ye first the kingdom of nature that the kingdom of man might be realized.

(Unsoeld, 1976, p. 4)

I was at Rumney Cliffs, one of my favorite rock-climbing areas in New Hampshire. I was on a climb that required almost all my current capabilities. When I can "pull it off," it gives me tremendous feelings of reenergizing and revitalization. When I am engaged in this adventure experience, I don't intend to apply much of this to my future beyond the hour or so I bask in my self-satisfaction. My interaction with this experience is full. I live for the climb in the moment and the tremendous feelings it gives me during and immediately after the experience. However, at other times, I have utilized rock climbing as an adventure experience in a totally different manner. For example, I have:

- Structured rock-climbing experiences to teach others how to become better instructors of rock-climbing;
- Facilitated rock climbing experiences with corporate executives to support more collaborative and risk-taking behaviors when appropriate in their business practices; and
- Conducted family therapy with families who have an adolescent facing identified social-emotional issues that need to be addressed.

In these situations, the purpose of rock climbing became more than the reenergizing or revitalization of a recreational experience. For these groups, the value of these experiences lay not in the recreational activity but in how the adventure experience created positive, productive, or functional lasting changes for the clients. As demonstrated in the quote above by Unsoeld (1976) in one of his most moving speeches on the spiritual values of the wilderness, he reminds us that we intentionally choose to go into adventure/wilderness settings to experience valuable lessons and then focus on co-creating with clients beneficial and lasting dynamics of change. These dynamics aid clients in learning, behaving, and changing, empowering them to return to the "regular world" and operate more effectively. Unsoeld holds us even further accountable by stating that if we can't bring the clients and this learning back to their "real world," we have failed.

Much of the confusion surrounding transfer principles may lie in the very center or purpose of a specific program and its targeted goals. In determining whether the transfer of learning/change is important to an adventure program, the answer lies in the very reason why you are adventuring! Adventure programs can have a wide variety of goals that can include recreation, educational objectives, corporate purposes, and therapeutic change (Priest & Gass, 2020). When adventure programs are used for creating enjoyable experiences or revitalizing/reenergizing participants with no lasting benefits from the experience and only to "live in the moment," then the future use of these adventure experiences, beyond the pictures and great memories, hold little value for the participant.

However, if the expectation is for the adventure program to produce educational, organizational/developmental, or therapeutic change for the client's future, then transfer of learning becomes imperative on both an effectiveness level and even an ethical one. Such a principle lies in the very fabric of adventure programming and shapes its central figures and core principles. Dewey (1938) informs us that one of the key principles of educative experiences is the ability for a learning experience to have a positive effect on future learning experiences. Dewey calls this the continuity of learning. This continuity is one of the two main criteria of learning. Without strong continuity from one learning experience to another, learning becomes miseducative and "has the effect of arresting or distorting the growth of future experience" (p. 25). Dewey goes further to state that without continuity in learning experiences, education is "defective" (p. 27), "unworthy" (p. 33), and "retards growth" (p. 36).

Finally, the teachings of Marina Ewald and Kurt Hahn confirm the definitive separation between these goals of adventure programming. Hahn was well known for his quotations about teaching "through the sea, not for the sea" in the early establishment of Outward Bound. Adapting Hahn's quotation to my rock-climbing example, Hahn's ideology and pragmatic maxim would stress the purpose of rock-climbing *not for teaching people to be better rock climbers, but for using rock climbing to teach people to be better people.* The purpose of adventure experiences, for Hahn, is as medium or process rather than outcome or product. Some therapists have misunderstood the role of transfer in adventure programming by envisioning it as an outcome/product not a medium/process.

Research on transfer and facilitation in adventure programming

> *Yet there is little empirical evidence to back up the belief in the efficacy of transfer generally, let alone as a central OAE (outdoor adventure education) concept...there is a lack of convincing evidence that long term transfer occurs.*
>
> (Brown, 2010, p. 19)

In his article portraying transfer as the "Achilles' heel" of outdoor adventure education, Brown (2010) asks, "where is the evidence that one generation of facilitation is more affected than others in promoting transfer?" (p. 14). Unfortunately, almost all elements of the outdoor adventure education field lack evidence. Within the OAE field, however, the research on facilitation is probably much more complete than in other areas in the field. The following is a summary illustrating research areas on facilitation and transfer in the outdoor adventure programming field.

Historically speaking, the first few examinations studying the differences in outcomes with various facilitation styles failed to find any statistically significant differences. In looking at the differences between facilitation styles with couples participating in an adventure enrichment program, Gillis (1986) found no significant differences in couples that participated in programs with metaphorically framed experiences when compared to participants not receiving metaphorically framed experiences. MacRea et al. (1993) examined the use of a one-day, high-ropes-only training course for firefighters on developing positive risk-taking propensity. This study used a randomized comparison group design with the control group not receiving the ropes course experience and the treatment group receiving the ropes course training experience. This treatment group was further divided in half through random assignment to a group receiving just the adventure experience, and the other group receiving the adventure experience with metaphoric framing. While the overall treatment group showed significantly different positive gains in risk-taking propensity, no significant difference was found between the group receiving metaphor framing with their adventure experience and the group receiving just the adventure training experience. While no significance was found in either of these studies and comparing facilitation styles, both authors stated in their conclusions that if modifications for presenting metaphoric introductions could be improved, their changes might result in different findings.

Taking heed of the advice from Gillis and Priest, Doherty (1995) designed a study to examine the differences between metaphoric framing (fifth generation facilitation – metaphoric model), post experience debriefing (third generation facilitation – Outward Bound Plus), and no facilitation (first generation facilitation – mountains speak for themselves). She conducted a one-day ropes course experience for university residence assistants in the United States. Metaphors created for the fifth level of facilitation followed the model structure presented by Gass (1990) and illustrated further by Hirsch and Gillis (2004). Eighty-four (84) resident assistants (RAs) participated in the study and were divided into one of these three groups. Each group's potential changes in team-building were measured immediately prior to the challenge course experience ("pretest"), immediately after the experience ("acquisition"), and 30 days following the training program ("retention"). The instrument used to measure changes was an adapted version of the Group Environmental Scale (GES) (Moos & Humphrey, 1974), a measurement tool designed to assess the social-environmental characteristics and changes of small groups.

In the most expansive and rigorous yet similar study with European corporate executives working on teamwork in the workplace, Gass and Priest (2006) examined changes in facilitation styles, measuring not only *what* was offered in terms of facilitation but also *when* it occurred. Four intact work groups from four regional head offices received a corporate adventure training program with four different styles of facilitation: (1) no metaphoric framing or debriefing associated with the training, (2) metaphoric debriefing following each training exercise, (3) metaphoric framing preceding the training experience, and (4) metaphoric framing before and debriefing after the training experience. A fifth group acted as a control group and received no teamwork program.

The 72-hour residential program began with goal setting and socialization, continued with group initiatives, and ended with action planning and closure experiences. All five groups were identical in composition and structure with one regional vice-president, three divisional directors, and 19 departmental managers. Each group's level of teamwork was measured one month before, one month after, six months after, and 12 months following the program.

As shown in the graph in Figure 9.1, all four groups showed significant increase in teamwork over the two-month period measured before and after the training program. Teamwork for the control group did not change over the study period, indicating changes experienced by the other four groups were likely due to the facilitation technique and training program they received rather than other influences occurring at the time.

Initial changes: The group receiving both the metaphoric framing and debriefing possessed the greatest initial and statistically significant increases in teamwork scores and the group with no framing or debriefing experienced the least (yet still significant) increases in teamwork scores. The groups receiving either the metaphoric framing or debriefing had similar initial increases in teamwork, but these gains were moderate compared to those of the group receiving both forms of facilitation.

Maintenance changes: In terms of maintaining teamwork levels, all groups showed significant decreases, likely due to the lack of follow-up procedures implemented to support the groups in their efforts to apply

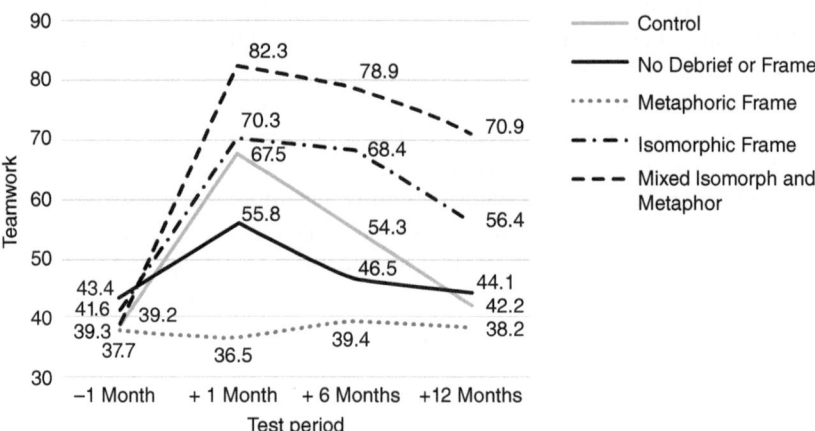

Figure 9.1 Changes in mean index scores for the (TDI-m) over a one-year study

new behaviors back at work. Teamwork levels for the no framing or debriefing group regressed to near baseline after six months. The metaphoric debriefing group's teamwork also returned to baseline levels after 12 months. The metaphoric framing group's teamwork remained elevated for six months, but then levels dropped significantly at 12 months yet remained higher than baseline. Teamwork levels for the metaphoric framing and debriefing group also remained elevated after six months and remained higher than for any of the other groups after 12 months.

Regarding the transfer of learning, this randomized control designed study showed that not only did the transfer of learning occur from adventure experience, but also that the *type* of properly executed facilitation also made a difference in both initial and maintenance levels of transfer. Such long-term positive transfer effects have been demonstrated not only in quantitative studies, but also qualitative studies (Gass, Garvey, & Sugerman, 2003).

Further evidence of facilitation differences with transfer has been shown in recent studies with juvenile offenders and juvenile sex offenders. Gillis, Gass, and Russell (2008) reported statistically significant differences with juvenile offender re-arrest rates after one, two, and three years between an adventure-based behavior management program (BMtA), an outdoor therapeutic camping (no facilitation) comparison group (OTC), and the standard Youth Development Center (YDC) non-adventure group in the State of Georgia. As seen in Figure 9.2, the

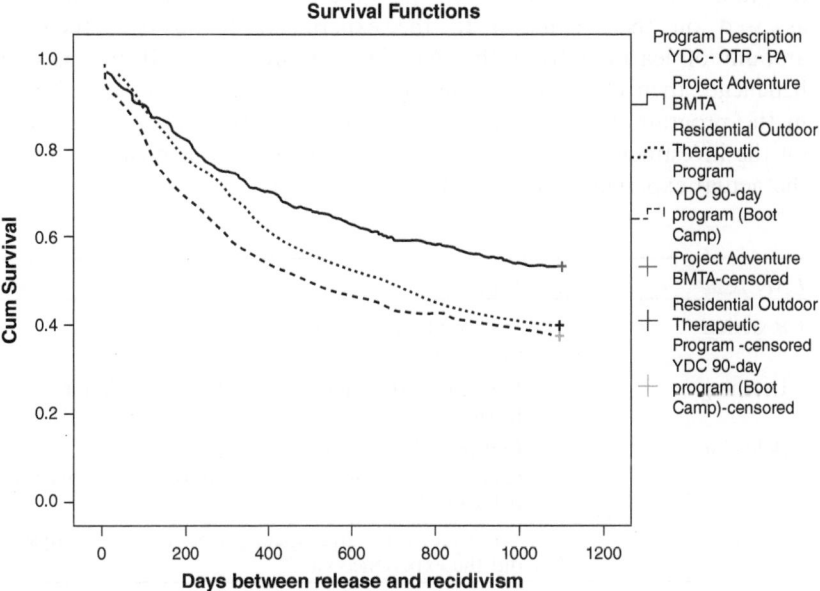

Figure 9.2 Days between release and recidivism

differences between the facilitated adventure group (BMtA) and the OTC and YDC groups grew even larger with time.

Gillis and Gass (2010) found similar statistically significant findings with the comparison of an adventure-based behavior management program for juvenile sex offenders (i.e., LEGACY), traditional treatment-as-usual program (i.e., YDC), and other specialized programs (OSP). The findings of empirically evidenced long-term transfer in these studies directly answer Brown's (2010) question "...where is the evidence that one generation (i.e., type, form, style) of facilitation is more effective than others in promoting transfer?" (p. 14).

There has been an increase in the expectation for evidence-based adventure programming. Programs that present themselves as working effectively with a particular client group should be accountable for meeting these expectations. As stated earlier, if the client is enjoying a recreational experience for recreational purposes, then the adventure program has met its contracted objective. However, if a client engages in rock climbing for educational, developmental, or therapeutic reasons and does not experience the transfer of change/contracted benefit from the experience, then the professionals of the adventure program should reexamine their program goals.

Kirkpatrick (1994) presents a very workable model representing one way of linking together different forms of evaluating program effectiveness that mesh well with outcomes related to transfer of learning. In this model, Kirkpatrick moves through a logical sequence of evaluating program effectiveness. As seen in Figure 9.2 participants are first assessed on their reaction to the experience. If positive, then the amount of learning from the experience is evaluated. If this level is beneficial, then changes in behavior occurring because of participation in the program are evaluated. If this level is successful, then a return on the investment of the program's cost is measured against the cost of the actual experience provided by the program.

Level Issue	Question Answered	Sample Tool
1 Reaction	How well did they enjoy the experience?	Rating Sheets
2 Learning	How much did they learn?	Tests, Simulations
3 Behavior	Did the experience result in changes in targeted behaviors?	Outcomes Performance Measures
4 Results	What return on investment did the experience yield?	Cost-Benefit Analysis

This model represents one way the transfer of learning takes on an ever-increasing importance for a program. Recreational programs are interested in providing enjoyable experiences for participants. They commonly use program evaluation sheets that ask participants if they found the experience enjoyable and what might be done in the future to make it even more so. As explained earlier, transfer of learning typically takes on little relative importance for the client or the program at this level. However, as programs become involved in adventure therapy and are held accountable to its outcome expectations of learning, behavior, and results, transfer of learning takes on greater importance. For example, certain approaches (e. g., boot camps, "Scared Straight" programs) with delinquent youth have not only failed to work but, in some cases, have indoctrinated youth to greater levels of delinquency behavior (Level 3) (i.e., negative transfer) and have also cost taxpayers four times more than traditional adjudication techniques (Level 4) (e.g., residential incarceration facilities). In one study, Gillis and Gass (2009) examined the treatment outcomes for the Legacy Program in Georgia using Project Adventure's BMtA model with juvenile sex offenders. It showed significant treatment effectiveness in rearrest rates when compared to youth development centers and other specialized programs. The Program's effectiveness continued after one, two, and three years post-treatment. This level of expectation regarding transfer and related evaluation speaks directly to the "...linking of programming in the outdoors and the livelihood of outdoor educators" (Brown, 2010, p. 14) conducting such programs.

10 Adventure therapy experiences

In this chapter, 24 adventure therapy activities are presented. They illustrate how adventure therapy can be used as an experiential therapeutic tool. The five basic underpinnings that foster therapeutic benefits for these activities include: (1) Experiential centered change, (2) Immersion into nature, (3) Enriched group process, (4) Challenging experiences, and (5) Use of metaphor. In the chapter, the activities are categorized to assist therapists in activity selection. Some of these categories include assessment, treatment, group size, and type of metaphoric transfer.

Metaphors are used in three ways. The first is spontaneous metaphoric transfer. This is where the linking of the adventure experience and the client's issue naturally match one another during an experience. The second is analogous metaphoric experiences which is when the client makes a metaphoric connection during the debriefing. The third is structured metaphoric transfer and this is when the therapist proactively "sets the stage during the activity" for the client to make a connection.

#1. Back-to-back

Therapeutic approach

In their efforts to change, clients will sometimes try first to change externally when really what is needed is internal change. For example, clients often try to perform superficial and physical changes that are externally recognizable when internal changes might serve the client better.

One of the dynamics reinforcing this issue is that external change is often much easier and more immediate to observe and recognize than internal changes. Sometimes, difficulties can arise when the internalization and self-education of clients in their change processes are required for long-lasting change. This activity highlights these points/issues for the client and individuals connected to or associated with the client (e.g., family members).

For whom: Partners/couples: adults, children. Two clients to an infinite number of paired-up individuals

Set-up and needs: None. Clients are standing facing each other.

DOI: 10.4324/9781032640303-10

Therapeutic Experiential Activity	Assessment	Treatment	Equipment	Estimated Time Needed (minutes)	Individual, Partners, or Group	Metaphoric Transfer: Spontaneous Analogous Structural
Back-to-Back	Y	Y	None	15-30	P, G	Sp, An, St
Balancing Tree	Y	Y	Blindfolds	15-30	I	Sp, An, St
Circles in the Air	Y	Y	None	10-15	I	An, St
Compliment the Masterpiece	Y	Y	Diff. colored crayons, paper	15-45	P	An, St
Don't Touch Me	Y	Y	Hula Hoop	15-30	G	St
Embrace Change	Y	Y	None	15-20	I, P, G	An, St
Family Sculpting	Y	Y	None	30-45	G	An
Finding Solutions	Y	Y	Objects, Blindfolds	15-30	P	Sp, An, St
Give Me 10	N	Y	None	10-20	G	An
Handling What You've Got	Y	Y	None	5-15	I	Sp, An, St
Hands Down	N	Y	None	15-30	G	An, St
Helium Loop	Y	Y	Hula Hoop	15-30	G	Sp, An, St
Key on the Wise Guide	N	Y	Sturdy chairs, Blindfolds	15-30	G	Sp, An, St
Paper Drop	Y	Y	Paper	15-30	G	An
Parents' (Caregivers') Quality Call	Y	Y	Blindfolds	10-20	P	An
Path to Recovery	N	Y	50 feet cord, trees/posts, Blindfolds	30-45	G	Sp, An, St
Play Together-Stay Together	Y	Y	None	15-30	P	Sp, An, St
Scarf Pull	Y	Y	Scarf	10-20	I	Sp, An, St
Stepping Stones	N	Y	Objects, Blindfolds	30-45	G	An, St
The System	Y	Y	Paper cups, Bandanas, water source or beans	20-40	G	An, St
Turning Over a New Leaf	Y	Y	Tarp	15-30	G	An, St
Warp Speed	Y	Y	Catchable objects	10-20	G	Sp, An, St
Wrestling With Conflict	Y	Y	None	10-20	P	An, St
You Cup Has Holes!	Y	Y	Paper cups, Pencils, water/beans	15-30	G, P, I	Sp, An

Figure 10.1 Various characteristics of experiential therapeutic activities

Facilitation

Paired individuals begin by standing facing each other and deciding who will "go first." (If you have a client who is working on a particular change process, this person should be the person who goes first.) When the therapist tells them to "go," they will turn around back-to-back without touching. The person who is going first ("the changer") must change three things on their body (in 15–25 seconds). The therapist tells them to turn around, and the person who did not change things ("guesser") tries to figure out what is different with the person (15 seconds). The "changer" will verify their guesses. I ask if there are any questions and if not, I have the individuals turn back-to-back and repeat this procedure again.

After the second round is completed, I ask for some quick observations as to how easy it was for individuals to change things, what were some of the things changed, and how easy it was to guess the changes. Following this brief input, the two individuals are asked to turn back-to-back immediately, and the "changer" is asked to change three additional (new) things about themselves in the next 15–25 seconds. After this time, individuals again turn and face one another, and the observer tries to guess the three new changes. The same verification/question process occurs for a third time in the same roles.

As clients progress through the three rounds, the changes typically remain external but become more difficult to accomplish (i.e., people start running out of ideas on what to change). People start looking for assistance to develop items to change, and observers become more skilled in recognizing the changes. The therapist's goal is to use questions to help clients find parallel structures between the activity and their reality (e.g., a parent is the guesser, the child is the changer because the parent observes the changes of the child and the child is often the one giving information.).

After relevant and appropriate discussion, the clients are again asked to go back-to-back for another round of changes. If the client making changes has yet to perform any internal changes, they must attempt to do so in this round. Sometimes, clients ask for guidance on what to change or what internal change means. The therapist explains what clients have changed so far externally in therapy to help them understand internal change. Following this, the therapist asks what examples of internal change might be relevant to them. This discussion can be done privately or with other clients. After agreeing upon one or two examples, the therapist invites the client and their observer to stand back-to-back and go again. It usually takes more work for the client to show internal change and for the observer to recognize it. Clients and observers once again complete three rounds of changes When appropriate roles can be switched in the partnerships.

Debrief

Several learnings can occur. Some of the most common include:

- External change is usually much easier than internal change
- External change is usually the first form of change attempted by clients
- External change is usually the easiest to observe
- External change usually takes less investment and commitment

Again, the length of debriefing will vary with the purpose of the experience (see treatment applications below). If done for just a brief bit of insight, having people share their responses throughout the activity can usually result in reaching the objective of the experience. If greater depth is desired, asking questions about the parallel processes between this activity and clients' reality/concepts/feelings about change issues will take much more time.

Treatment applications

There are many potential applications for this activity to be tailored around the specific needs of a client group. When working with a particular group structure like a family, I will assign individuals tasks and roles congruent with their family structure (e.g., an adolescent being the person changing and parents being the observers of change). Sometimes, to build empathy in the therapeutic moment, I will reverse the roles of these clients.

#2. Balancing tree

Therapeutic application

Clients sometimes struggle to find appropriate levels of balance in their lives. Increasing their understanding through experience with reflection, as described here, can provide insights into how they can maintain or create balance in their lives. Such experiences can also show how current imbalanced conditions or positions create unhealthy states of being that must be changed to achieve a healthier, more desirable state.

For whom: Adults, children

Set-up and needs: Open space, flat objects (e.g., paper plate, small book), blindfolds (optional)

Facilitation

Invite the group into a circle or face an individual client. Ask them to focus on a fixed point well off in the distance. While maintaining a strong and clear focus on this fixed point, ask them to lift their right foot off the ground and hold it there while maintaining their balance on their left foot alone. For some groups or individuals, you can have them go into the yoga "tree stance position," where their right foot is placed inside their left thigh, and both hands are fully extended above their head.

After a brief evaluation of how they did, have the client close their eyes while standing still with both feet solidly on the ground. As they did previously, ask them to lift their right foot off the ground or move into the yoga tree position.

Again, the goal is to maintain balance and not place the right foot down. After 30 seconds, have them plant their right foot firmly back on the ground.

For their third task, remind them to direct their gaze to the focus spot and ask them to extend their arms out to their sides with their palms facing up. Have them place an object (book, rock) in each palm and on top of their head to see if they can also balance these things. Ask them to lift their foot again while keeping the objects in place. Give 30 seconds or so for this, and if participants drop an object or stumble, reassure them. After completing this, invite the client to do this "balancing act" with their eyes closed.

Debrief

As with most experiential/adventure experiences, therapists examine and utilize what themes emerge from client behaviors and dialogue. One of the concepts used in this activity is creating a kinesthetic experience where balancing with a clear focus on an intended goal/object is more easily achieved when looking at a focus spot than when no focus or intention exits. This is commonly true when clients are "weighed down" or attempting to balance other objects/objectives at the same time as themselves. To facilitate these concepts, as well as additional objectives, a common set of questions may include the following:

- Was there a difference in your ability to balance between the first and second rounds? Their third and fourth rounds?
- What type of conditions created the differences in these experiences?
- How might such differences relate to your perspectives and life?
- Is there anything they could imagine doing to make this challenge easier? If so, what? (Try out clients' ideas.)
- How might such changes relate to issues of balance in their life?

The metaphor of seeing clearly and with focus can be utilized to explain how maintaining balance sometimes leads to seeing the situation more clearly. Once the imbalance can be seen and experienced, new ways of being (include client suggestions) can be applied to the new situation. For example, if the client says, "Well, if I could just hold onto something (chair, wall, you), it would be easier." Such an answer may open a valuable examination of who/what we lean on when we become imbalanced. Another example may be if the client asks you to hold some of the objects or wants to place them all in one hand.

Contraindications

The use of blindfolds can be traumatic for clients with power and control issues. Offer the option of simply closing one's eyes, allowing the client to maintain more control.

#3. Circles in the air

Therapeutic application

This activity focuses on understanding the role that perspective has in determining a person's perspective. In addition, how a client can learn to appreciate other people's perspectives and how it can affect their reality. This activity could also bring awareness to the abilities and challenges every person holds.

For whom: Individuals: adults, children from one to unlimited

Set-up and needs: Standing space – no movement, no props

Facilitation

Ask clients to point one of their index fingers up in the air. Imagine that there is a clock looking down at you. With the pointed finger draw a circle clockwise around the imaginary clock. Continue to draw continuous circles as you bring your finger in front of your face and then down to your waist. Now notice the direction that your circles are going. Are the circles going clockwise or counterclockwise when at your waist? Clients may seem confused so suggest that they try it again with the emphasis of going clockwise when looking up in the air.

Debrief

Immediately after the second round ask clients to share what happened. Note that you will probably have several different responses. Then ask how it happened that some people's finger supposedly changed direction and others said it didn't. Consider having partners share this together first and then out to the group. One response that tends to emerge is that the perspective taken will lead to a clockwise or counterclockwise response.

You can also discuss how a person's perspective affects their understanding and behaviors. In addition, how one person's perspective affects the beliefs or actions taken by another person. Share the possibility that one experience for a person can create different interpretations by that person.

#4. Compliment the masterpiece

Therapeutic approach

The experience of being a part of a group or dyad with individuals who have different opinions, perspectives, cultural norms, and approaches is one that we all must learn to navigate. Working in tandem with others is essential to human relationships and requires self-awareness and perspective-taking skills. If a client struggles to see the strengths within another's approach or perspective, they may present as being quite rigid or judgmental, as someone unable to build a working relationship or appreciate the contributions of others who are different from themselves. It could be that a client needs help seeing how they can work with another individual with whom they feel inherently in conflict. It could also be that a client would benefit from working on how they contribute to a group in a complementary way. Asserting appropriate boundaries while respecting others' boundaries is a vital part of this. This activity allows clients to take on different roles in a co-creative process to explore these concepts.

For whom: Partners/Couples; adults, children

Set-up and needs: Space to draw, different colored crayons, & a sheet of paper for each partnership

Facilitation

In this activity, you will make a visible product that illustrates how complementary parts come together to create a masterpiece. The best way to frame this may be as a fun way to see how people interact with one another when being creative. For this activity, individuals pair up and are given a piece of paper, two different colored crayons, and a flat surface for drawing. When the therapist says "Go!" each person draws a squiggle on their paper. When they hear "Stop!" they put down the crayon. Ask the clients to exchange squiggle drawings. Then, invite clients to use their crayon to create a simple "picture" using the newly acquired squiggle. Now, ask partners to share their drawings with each other. If you have extra time, ask pairs to create a story for their picture. If the group is of a reasonable size allow pairs to share their drawings.

Debrief

This activity can guide people struggling to coexist with others in a fluid, healthy manner, examining their attitudes and behaviors in a non-threatening way. It is rich for debriefing along themes of sharing, control, letting go, and appreciating and acknowledging the contribution of others. I would frame the debrief with specific questions and observations and then expand to conceptual or applied questions.

- How did it feel to make your first squiggle? Did you have an idea formed in your mind of what the picture might become?
- What did you think when you got the squiggle from your partner? How did you decide what to draw?
- Once you began drawing, was it easy or hard to incorporate the original squiggle? Why, or why not?

- Did you speak to each other while drawing? If so, what did you talk about?
- How much did you let the original squiggle guide your drawing? What was this like (easy, challenging, fun...)?
- What did you notice about how your partner utilized your squiggle?
- What is one thing you really like about your partner's drawing?
- What is one thing you might have done differently during this activity?
- How does the way you contribute and interact with your partner resemble how you are at home with your family, friends, etc.?
- What things helped you to complete this activity that might also help you with a future interaction?

Therapeutic applications

As mentioned in the facilitation and debrief sections, this activity can be successfully applied to several different populations and sets of issues. Some of these applications and issues can include:

- Couples as an early assessment activity
- Individuals struggling with identity differentiation and healthy independence
- To enhance communication and creativity within a relatively functional family
- Adolescents/young adults who are looking for autonomy from a parent(s)
- Adult/child pairs who are struggling with trust, power, boundaries, etc.

Contraindications: None, just awareness of young children using crayons
   Source: Inspired by "Partnered Squiggle" in Lung et al. (2008). Thank you, Maurie, for creating this activity!

#5. Don't touch me

Therapeutic application

This case study and subsequent prescriptive activity originated from working with a social worker in Taiwan who asked if there was an adventure experience to use in assisting a young female client who had been sexually assaulted by a community member. This situation was steeped with issues of blame and misdirected accusations. These issues presented themselves as overwhelming feelings of guilt (i.e., blaming herself that the sexual abuse incident was her fault) combined with her family's and community's perceptions that she must have done something to "attract" or "deserve" the perpetration. (Note: It is not uncommon for victims to internalize this belief system and support the systems that sometimes reinforce these beliefs of blame.) This activity was offered and designed to assist this client in shifting the focus of blame from herself to her attacker and redirecting the focus of the social system toward her abuser. Some suggestions include:

- Provide an initial parallel structure of what occurred yet restructure the solution of the adventure experience to mirror, bring to the discussion, and support positive changes in the client's and her community's belief systems.
- In this parallel structure, reframe the interpretation of what happened to the victim for her to see that it is not her fault to be sexually assaulted.
- Emphasize the need for community/family members' contribution to making the environment safe for all the community/family members.

For whom: Group: adults, adolescents

Set-up and needs: Have all group members stand in a circle facing each other. Have two group members grasp a hula-hoop approximately one meter in diameter with their hands, and then have the remaining members join hands. The group must work together to pass each of their bodies through the hula-hoop without letting go of each other's hands and without the hoop touching anyone in the group (other than the two individuals holding the loop). The holders also need to go through the hula-hoop without touching it except for the hands holding onto the hoop. Using a segmented hula-hoop is encouraged because it allows versatility in making the activity easier or more difficult according to the client's needs.

Facilitation

"The goal of this activity is to have all of you go through the hoop without touching it. When doing this activity, taking care of yourself and one another can be incredibly important, in some ways a lot like taking care of family/community members. So please pay close attention to what helped you to go through the hoop. What are some ways your family/community takes care of one another?" (Common answers can be: *"We look after/watch out for one another by...,"* *"We care for one another by ..."* As a facilitator, you are looking for clarity and ownership of client responses, for these often are the seeds of change you will present back to clients throughout the exercise and during the discussion following the experience). *"I encourage you to consider using some of these concepts in this next activity."*

Clients begin the activity by passing one another through the hula-hoop. While it does depend upon the family/community, I usually do not "call" the touches of the hula-hoop when I see them and leave this up to the group. This can be a rich point of discussion in the debriefing if clients do not say anything and "keep secrets." The activity progresses until someone touches the hula-hoop.

Depending upon the group and the behaviors and comments they present, the following questions may serve to provide rich sources of metaphoric connections to the presenting issue:

- How did the person touch?
- Whose fault was it?
- How come the touch happened?
- How vigilant were you as a group in monitoring touches? Did that make a difference?
- When you were successful, what were you doing? Did anything change to stop your success?

For an interesting dynamic, you can ask each group member to say, "Don't touch me" as they pass through the hoop. This can sometimes add "richness" between what people say and what occurs in physical actions. It is interesting to note the congruity or incongruity levels between this request/words and actions. For some groups, this can be a rich point of discussion.

The center of many discussions is that the group finds itself much more functional if it stops blaming the person who touches the hula-hoop and develops a more systemic method for achieving the objective. It typically is much easier for most groups to have the person passing through the hoop work *with* the group rather than have the person do it all themselves and the group pay little to no attention to their efforts.

Again, using a hula-hoop with multiple/separate sections can be beneficial. By choosing this kind of hula-hoop, the facilitator can take out pieces when needed to present the appropriate level of challenge. This also has the metaphorical benefit of connecting to the reality.

Debrief

Debriefings can cover a variety of topic areas, but the most common themes that arise are: (1) it is easy to blame the person who touches the hula hoop, but quite often it is not the fault of this individual; (2) the success of the group is highly related to the level of group collaborative effort; and (3) how these dynamics are related to issues of sexual abuse.

I then asked the group how realistic it was for everyone to be successful by doing the initiative themselves. One of the group members mentioned that it was impossible because there were too many blind spots for the person to see. This observation shifted the "blame structure" toward the attacker and not the victim. It also led to a discussion of how the group could increase its efforts to protect vulnerable individuals from future abuses.

#6. Embrace change (Folded arms)

Therapeutic application

Sometimes, the very thought or process of change can be enough to stimulate a significant degree of resistance in clients. Demystifying such a process can go a long way in reducing such resistance and enhancing the possibility of change. Sometimes words and language just don't provide:

- Enough awareness/motivation/understanding/foresight
- Proper pathways/methods to achieve enough reduction of resistance
- Encouragement for clients to embrace qualities associated with change

There are many potential applications for this activity to be tailored around the specific needs of a client group. Three of these reasons include:

1   The client's willingness to engage in an activity that will show a better understanding of what change may be like
2   To "set the stage" with potentially unwilling or resistant clients with "seeds of interpretation and defusing resistance" (e.g., this activity begins the process of differentiating client productive and client resistant behavior)
3   When clients (or even other colleagues) have questions about what adventure therapy looks or even feels like and need a quick interpretation.

For whom: One to an infinite number of adolescents, adults
Set-up and needs: None

Facilitation

I begin the experience by letting clients know I will invite them to respond to how they feel about the next set of actions I will ask them to perform.

Often, at least one group member sits or stands with their arms folded, sometimes even suggesting a state of non-verbal resistance. I ask them to fold their arms or keep their arms folded. Then I ask them, "How does this feel? What words would you use to express that feeling?" While a mixture of answers will often present themselves, many responses revolve around how this position "makes them feel shut off from the world, comfortable, closed to change, resistant," etc. I also ask them that if they were to see a person in this type of position, what would such a position tell them regarding nonverbal behavior? Again, while various responses may result, most revolve around thoughts of being closed to change and "I dare you to ask me to do anything!"

I then ask the group to look down at their arms and refold them with the current arm on top placed on the bottom and the arm currently on the bottom placed on top of the other arm. I also ask that people hold it once they can get in this position and not switch back. During this time, I quickly scan the group to find a representative sample of individuals having difficulty getting into this position, being uncomfortable in this position, and those individuals who are unable or unwilling to remain in this position for any length of time. After approximately five to ten seconds, I ask them again, "How does this feel? And what words would you use to express this feeling?" I often will scan back to individuals I see having difficulty or uncomfortableness with this new position and seek their answers. Responses often include being uncomfortable, wanting to change back, weird, different, new, and "I never felt that way before!" After soliciting several responses, I give "permission" for people to drop their arms or return to having them folded in the familiar way.

Debrief

The length of debriefing will vary with the purpose of the experience. If done for just a brief bit of insight, having people share their responses with one another can usually result in reaching the objective of the experience. If greater depth is desired, asking questions about the parallel processes between this activity and clients' perspectives about change issues will take much more time.

#7. Family sculpting

Therapeutic application

Family sculpting is a diagnostic and therapeutic technique first championed by Virginia Satir in the late 1960s. With well-grounded beginnings in Gestalt therapy, it offers active, experiential, and insightful perspectives that can provide some of the most influential forms of therapy. While there are many forms and techniques of family sculpting, its foremost technique is the way therapists approach young children in their assessment of the family. Family sculpting is used to help identify and work through dynamics contributing to unhealthy communication and challenges that may or may not be apparent to family members (Mason, 2010). Some of the major concepts that belong to therapists using family sculpture include the nonverbal visualization technique, the relational balance of individual group members, the representation of the coalition concept, and the structures of the family and its hierarchy.

For whom: Primarily for families, can be modified for therapeutic groups
Set-up and needs: None

Facilitation

Gather the family in an open space wide enough to move around. The therapist selects a family member to be the sculptor. Ideally, the person selected should possess a perceived critical role for the therapeutic process (e. g., the person with the most perceived power, the person who is identified as the "problem"). This person is invited to "sculpt" or position the members of the family that depicts their perception of the family's structure (e.g., emotional closeness, distance, alliances). In the sculpting process, the sculptor provides information about everyone so that the people playing the roles will understand what their character might say and how they might act.

Ask the family if anyone would have done this differently, and if so, why.

The therapist guides the family to make comments that are uninterrupted, open to hear from all members, and respected language. Members take turns being the sculpture and giving their representation of the family followed by a balanced debrief.

Debrief

The therapist begins the activity by having family members go around and state how they felt about each person. The therapist may also ask the sculptor to ask family members to share the thoughts they had before, during, and after a critical event (e.g., a tragic incident). The sculptor determines all details and positions of the participants, starting by asking the sculptor to recruit families before, during, and after a critical event.

- What surprised you about this session?
- Did you learn anything about yourself or other members of your family?
- Why did you arrange this member in relation to other members in the context of posture, space, and attitude?

#8. Finding solutions (Minefield)

Therapeutic application

This activity is designed for clients with substance abuse. The therapist creates the experience by designing an "obstacle style" course out of available objects that represent "problem" obstacles as well as potential solutions. Note this can be done with or without the assistance of clients, depending upon what makes best "therapeutic sense." Inside an office therapists can use chairs, tables, or other objects that can be bumped into gently without breaking. If you are outside things like trees and bushes or other elements of the natural landscape can be used. Better yet, encourage therapists to use metaphorically linked obstacles with clients, (e.g., symbolic problems like baggies filled with oregano or white flour; symbolic solutions like a phone to call their sponsor or an AA Big Book).

Once consequences for bumping into obstacles have been established, you can begin. The client might have a goal of getting to the other side quickly but doesn't follow the verbal cues and finds them bumping into

uickly. If the client is not able to adjust to new strategies
s proving to be difficult, a reframing of the rules and the
:ters) of the activity should be adjusted to help the client
ough working on their issues.
rtners/couples; adults, older children

Set-up and needs: Open space, objects to use as obstacles. Blindfold for
one partner

Facilitation

After constructing the obstacle course and the changing the placements, the clients begin the activity at one end of the obstacle course. Clients are in pairs with
consideration given to match up clients to their sponsors (e.g., AA sponsors,
supportive person). This activity typically involves blindfolding the client (if not
contraindicated), as the goal is for the client to move from one end of the
obstacle course to the other without encountering an obstacle. Clients may also
pick up resources (e.g., The Big Book, phone number of supportive person) as
they cross and carry it with them. It is the sponsor's job to guide the client verbally, but they remain still at the starting point. If the client hits an obstacle, they
must return to the beginning by looking and walking back to their sponsor and
begin again blindfolded. However, if a client has acquired at least one resource
(e.g., The Big Book) they can use it as a "pass" to be able to keep on crossing.

The rules for bumping into an obstacle should be framed to the life-
scenario that a client is currently dealing with. Clear penalties can be co-
created by the client and facilitator after the first try. Usually this helps
clients to take ownership of the activity. Some other suggestions for consequences for hitting an obstacle could be a delay of five seconds or a
question pertaining to problem solving in the client's real life.

Debrief

Participants should be careful when choosing their guide or voice in this
activity. Discussing what they look for in a guiding force to maneuver
them through the obstacle course could be an interesting way to look at
this activity. Another way to debrief would be to have the client identify
the obstacles in their life and name each before they start. They could also
choose to name who their guides are in the outside world.

Contraindications: Anyone made uncomfortable by blindfolds

#9. Give me 10

Therapeutic application

This intervention utilizes competition-based tasks to simulate a high-pressure
environment where clients can practice emotional regulation and patience. It

can be useful when working with clients with intermittent explosive disord.
as described below. You also can find a video of a role-play experience conducted by members of a workshop delivered at the International Association
for Experiential Education Conference in Montreal, Canada, in 2014. See:
https://www.youtube.com/watch?v=M0KsimKoNhg

For whom: Clients with intermittent explosive disorder (F63.81), i.e.,
impulsive or anger-based aggressive outbursts that have a rapid onset and
have little to no prodromal period. Outbursts typically last less than thirty
minutes and occur in response to minor provocation. Individuals often
have less severe episodes of verbal or non-damaging, non-destructive, non-
injurious physical assault between more severe episodes. Temper tantrums,
tirades, verbal fights, or assaults without damage can characterize
outbursts

Set-up and needs: Space to stand in a circle, no props

Facilitation

The therapists model the first round of the game to make sure everyone
understands how it is played. To begin the game, everyone stands in a circle
with one person in the center, and this person is "it," which means they are
the slapper (Tony). Begin with people in the circle stating their first name.
Every person in the circle puts their hands outstretched comfortably with
their palms facing up at their waist. The last person to say their name
(Chih-sing) begins the next round by stating the name of one person in the
circle (Irem). This same person (Irem) has to say the name of another
person in the circle before the person in the middle (Tony) slaps the hands of
the named person (Luis). If the person in the middle (Tony) slaps the hand
of the named person (Luis) before a circle person (Irem) says the name of a
new person, then the circle person is now in the middle. If the circle person
(Irem) can say the name of a new person (Andrés) before the middle person
does a slap, then the middle person (Tony) stays in the middle.

Debrief

- What were the most difficult times you had during the game? (e.g.,
  What was happening when you lost your temper/emotional?)
- Were there any times when you thought you would lose your temper,
  but it didn't happen? What did you do not to lose your temper?

#10. Handling what you've got (Homeostasis)

Therapeutic application

Client health is often determined by how they can maintain balance in
their lives through self-regulation and determination. The ability to handle

daily tasks, aligned with goals, can sometimes be appropriate and other times overwhelming. The capacity to prioritize, create functional systems, and determine what is necessary and desired in your lives (as well as what needs to be said "no" to) are all critical factors for maintaining a healthy homeostasis on a day-to-day basis.

For whom: Individuals: adults, children

Set-up and needs: Open space. Different unbreakable objects that can be held easily in a hand.

Facilitation

While this can be done with an individual client and a therapist serving as their partner, the activity will be described here with a group of clients working together in pairs. As with many adventure therapy experiences, this activity was probably preceded by client dialogue of situations matching the structure of the adventure experience. In this case, clients who take on more than they can handle become so overwhelmed that they lose their ability to hold onto any tasks.

In this case, the client ("Juan") presents strong and vivid images and descriptions of being overloaded with life tasks in daily experiences. Some of the client's expressions include comments such as "weighed down," "overwhelmed," "more than I can handle," "overburdened," etc. Such statements invite therapists to leave their chairs and use adventure experiences as a medium for change.

Utilizing this invitation with the language/reality the client presents, the therapist is symbolically representing the overloading process of Juan's behavior. For example, the therapist could say: "So, I heard you mention that you were taking on additional responsibilities at work. What is something you have that could remind you of your additional responsibilities at work." With this statement, the therapist places an object associated with work in the hands of the client. From this point, the therapist continues to put additional items into the client's hands, representing the collection of multiple things/ tasks the client had described to the therapist. This pattern of quickly adding objects continues until the client begins to drop things or utilizes a healthy coping mechanism (e.g., saying no or asking for help). Note that any of these answers provide a positive double-bind for the therapeutic session. On the one hand, if the client begins dropping things, this behavior enriches the therapeutic debriefing even further. If the client presents a healthy coping mechanism to handle the situation, the elements that led toward such behavior are debriefed and integrated into the client's life choices outside therapy.

Debrief

- How did you handle the additional elements of the process? Did you prioritize items and develop this strategy/plan for becoming more capable? Or was your plan spontaneous and not thought out very well?

- Was the process one where you could say no and balance capabilities with strategies?
- Is there any rule that could make this challenge easier? If so, what? Repeat the above, trying the client's ideas.

Contraindications: Clients should not be given extremely heavy objects where they could injure their back or other body parts

#11. Hands down

Therapeutic application

This activity focuses on maintaining a broad vision when trying to solve a problem. The goal for the clients is to guess a number between 0–10 based on the way I "roll" sticks from my hand onto the ground. As a therapist I make it appear that the number is determined by the way the sticks lay. However, unbeknown to the clients, the number for each round is determined by the number of fingers displayed.

This is a great activity to do with groups, particularly with groups who have clients with varying levels of group involvement.

For whom: Small groups (6-15): adults, adolescents, children (can be intact families or not)

Set-up and needs: Standing or sitting space, small objects that can be "rolled" onto the ground and held in one hand

Facilitation

Have your clients stand or sit in a circle and as the therapist, stand or sit in front of them. Lay out a few things (no more than 10) on the ground (e. g., sticks, stones, M&M's). Ask your clients, "How many are there" while at the same time, make your fingers show a number about 2 feet (.5m) away. For example, if four sticks are rolled, the therapist might put down two fingers (e.g., "peace" sign). The clients will likely say "four" when the correct answer is the number of fingers you put out, which was "two." The number of items can sometimes match your "finger number" and sometimes not match.

Continue this activity until your clients catch on to the "trick/answer." If one client understands what is going on and the others do not yet understand, ask the client that understands not to share the answer. Conclude when all the clients "get it" or the activity is complete for some other reason.

Sample presentation: This activity might help clients who are working on black-and-white thinking, having trouble seeing multiple perspectives, or have tunnel vision and are inflexible when it comes to the things they want. Since the answers to the activity are "right in front of them," clients may experience feelings of frustration or incompetence before the "aha moment." This activity has the potential for fruitful debriefing and discussion.

Debrief

Areas for exploration during debriefing might include the clients' ability to think broadly and see multiple perspectives. Reflection questions for this activity include:

- How did you feel when you "got it?"
- How did the group dynamic shift as some people were able to figure out the activity while others were left still trying to understand the answer?
- Have you experienced these feelings in other areas of your life? If so, what was happening then that was like this activity?

Variations: You could ask if anyone who "got it" would like to be the person placing down the objects for additional playing.

#12. Helium stick

Therapeutic application

This is one of those wonderful activities where each person's success depends on their ability to see the interconnectedness among the group members. The systemic lessons that have occurred with groups who have done this activity have been some of the richest I have seen.

For whom: Groups of 6–12 adults, children
Set-up and needs: Open space for individuals to stand, a pole or stick (6–7 feet long, can be shorter if group is on the smaller size)

Facilitation

The goal of this activity is for participants to lower the hoop using only the back of their hands. Participants stand in two lines facing each other. They put their hands out in front with palms facing down. Each person's hands should alternate with the hands of the person across (like a "zipper"). Finally, participants close their hands, except for their forefinger (pointer), while keeping the "zipper." Tell participants that after the rules are explained, they will get into this position and begin. Every person must always maintain personal contact with their fingers on the pole/stick. If a person's finger slips off the pole/stick, the group starts again. Once the group understands these rules, I ask everyone to "zipper up."

Debrief

The pole/stick almost always rises due to some invisible force despite the concerted attempts to lower it to the ground. Many groups can only stop the pole/stick from moving once they think of the task beyond their individual responsibility and needs. The analogy is that the pole/stick will go to the ground only when the participants think of this activity as a system working together.

- Was it as easy as you thought it was?
- How did people's perceptions influence their behavior?
- What were significant incidences during the activity?
- What adjustments took place throughout the activity?

#13. Key on the wise guide

Therapeutic application

This case example uses an adventure experience as a medium for change with a woman from a disempowered background. In working with this woman, the activity was structured where she needed to sort through the multiple voices she was hearing about herself, finding and keying in on the good positive messages from her support group, and not listening to, or even quieting, the voices/messages of negativity in her life.

This adventure experience's therapeutic objective was to assist a woman feeling disempowered to change her area of focus, centering on the solutions in her life to help her bring about functional change. Associated with this process was the ability to screen out voices and sources of negativity that were a significant source of disempowerment. This woman was a single mother who presented herself as having a low level of internal locus of control, feelings of "being stuck," and little support from her family of origin.

For whom: Adolescents, adults. In addition an apropriate number of adults who will serve as spotters.

Set-ups and needs: A minimum of 6 very study, non-folding chairs (without arms) placed in a straight line in different directions, with an identified starting and ending point. If very study chairs are not available, "tree cookies" of a thickness of no more than 4 inches can be used. Each cookie should be large enough to accommodate two adult feet. Carpet remnants, cut into "circles" can also be used.

Also, you need one blindfold per partnership (unless contraindicated.)

Facilitation

At least six sturdy chairs need to be selected for this therapeutic initiative (unless tree "cookies" or carpet "circles" are warranted due to client physical capabilities or characteristics.). Prior to this activity, all clients need to be assigned a role. The therapist decides alone or in concert with the client group, who will take the role of "the person needing help" and who will take the role as "the wise guide." The "person needing help" will be standing on the seats of chairs as they move across the room. The "wise guide" will guide them across these chairs using only their voice. All other clients become spotters for the activity under the therapist's supervision. This activity is only conducted when clients have demonstrated they can spot appropriately. This activity begins with the "person needing help" (identified client) selecting a specific therapeutic goal that they will focus on during this activity (e.g., anxiety, self-confidence). This therapeutic goal is determined with the help of the therapist.

The room is set up with a line of sturdy, non-folding chairs (chairs touching one another in different configurations) in a pattern that goes from a starting to an ending point. The client ("the person needing help") will be invited to stand on the seats of the chairs and move to the end of the line of chairs. The "wise guide's" role is to guide the client ("the person needing help") from the first chair in the line, to the end by only using their voice. The guide provides directions and empowering statements about their therapeutic goal (e.g., "You know how to place your foot in the middle of the seat." "Center your thoughts on moving forward"). Other members in the group serve as spotters [i.e., knees slightly bent, "bumpers" (hands up)] and are "voices of negativity" (e.g., "You are not going to make it!") throughout the process. Once the client reaches the end of the line of chairs, they step down, remove their blindfold and debrief. The therapist then decides if another two clients will complete the activity.

Sample Presentation

The therapist to the client ("the person needing help") says, "It was great to listen to your story and hear aspects of your life that help or limit you from achieving your goals. This can be common with women who have worries about their future after a significant life change. The key for some women may lie in focusing on what will work rather than changing what doesn't work.

"After hearing your story, we would like to invite you to do an activity that could encourage you to listen to your inner voice. We know that this source of wisdom resides inside of you, but for some reason you cannot "hear" the positive messages. These wise messages are often mixed in with voices of negativity that can sometimes limit your potential. Your success in this activity, just like in your life, may be linked to your ability to reconnect to these wise messages as you screen out the negative messages that you may be hearing."

Debrief

The therapist debriefs the experience, focusing on issues pertinent to the client's reality. Some of the debriefing topics may center on:

• Negative voices coming from people who support the client

- The mixed messages that may occur in family systems
- What the client could do to be more successful
- Which part of the activity was most comfortable for the client
- What did the client do to make the hard parts easier.

It may also be insightful to label each chair as a specific obstacle for clients and metaphorically identify what enabled and empowered the client to reach and exceed that obstacle.

Contraindications

Allow individuals to close their eyes if they're unable to wear blindfolds. If individuals have ambulatory/physical challenges or their footwear is inappropriate (e.g., flip-flops).

#14. Paper drop

Therapeutic application

The activity asks clients to practice dealing with unexpected events and a changing environment. Communication, cooperation, special awareness, adaptability and team support are reinforced with this fun game.

For whom: Group of 3–20: adults, children

Set-up and needs: Space for the group to move. One piece of paper (letter size) for each group

Facilitation

Have the group stand in a circle. The participant in the middle holds the paper up, says another participant's name, and drops it. If the person whose name has been called catches the paper before it hits the ground, they choose another name and drop it again. If they fail to catch it, they must tear it in half before dropping it again. Participants are welcome to redefine the rules of the game: they can move around and even hand the paper to the person whose name they have called. This will allow the group to determine what level of risk they choose to engage in.

Debrief

In the debrief for this activity, it would be interesting to address the decisions people made, why they made them, and their effects on the other individuals in the group.

#15. Parents' (Caregivers') quality call

Therapeutic application

This activity can be used with various groups, but in this case, it was used with adults during a three-hour "couples only" session of a five-day family enrichment program. The initiative does not require extreme risk-taking, except for being unable to see because your eyes are closed and because of physical touch (which may be contraindicated for some participants). This is a good assessment activity for several things, some of which may include: (1) determining group members' ability to follow directions and take risks; (2) gathering an idea of the roles these individuals play in group settings; (3) observing each individual's comfort with conflict and frustration; (4) getting an idea of each individual's degree of comfort in working with other parents/caregivers as resources of information; and (5) examining how spouses work independently of one another.

The initiative, presented in this manner, emphasizes (1) what group members perceive as healthy attributes to be working on as parents/ caregivers and families; (2) the similarity of what parents/caregivers are looking for to make their families better than what they already are; (3) normalizing the interaction of parents/caregivers asking for help from other parents/caregivers in the group; (4) emphasizing that all families can use more of "something" to help be more functional; (5) increasing the level of sharing ideas among couples; and (6) having fun and setting the tone for fun during activities in this session as well as during the week.

For whom: Partners/caregivers

Set-up and needs: The setup for this initiative is much like the Hog Call initiative (Silver Bullets by Karl Rohnke, 1984, pp.98-99). Two therapists are required.

All proper safety issues should be followed (e.g., gentle, flat ground, no obstacles that could be run into or tripped on , reinforce the hands up "bumper" position, move at a safe, slow walking pace) and blindfolds (or eyes closed) for each person.

Facilitation

Parents/Caregivers are asked to "pair up" with someone they don't know well yet but who seems like someone they might want to seek out for parenting advice (not their partner/spouse). If there's an odd number of people (e.g., single parents/caregivers taking part in the program), one group can form a trio. After this is accomplished, have each pair or trio take five minutes to introduce themselves, Then each person decides one quality they seek to gain and share this quality with their partner. This quality doesn't have to be difficult for them, but may be a thing that, if they had more assistance, or just more of it, they would feel more capable as a parent/caregiver. In sharing this quality with their partner, each person should take approximately 30 seconds to describe the significance of this quality. They should not share this quality with other pairs at this time but should be reminded to remember their quality and their partner's quality.

After this, the pair decides who will be "it." All the "its" join hands with one therapist and close their eyes. The "not its" do the same with the other therapist.

Participants are told to keep their eyes closed while they are randomly distributed in the "playing area" and are asked not to move until they are directed to do so. The area should be large enough to move around but small enough for people to hear each other and the therapist. If client are unaware of the "bumpers up" position (i.e., hands up in front of chest), they should be taught this at the beginning of the activity.

Sample presentation

(Parents/caregivers are asked to stand in a circle) *"We'd like to do this activity that people find enjoyable and sometimes eye-opening. One of the things I'm aware of as a caregiver is that there are a lot of times that can be troublesome or worrying. It could be putting kids to sleep at night, potty training, juggling 15 things at once, having your child go out on their first date... Do you know what I mean? Can anyone share a time like this they've experienced?"* I look at others to share brief statements representing their projection of the parental/caregiving interactions they see as difficult.

"One of the things I know in dealing with these times is that certain qualities may be extremely important for me in my role as a parent/caregiver. It seems whenever I have these qualities, it makes things go so much easier and feel more competent as a parent/caregiver.

What we want you to do is think of one of these qualities, and when you have chosen the one that can be best represented by a single word, raise your right hand. This quality doesn't have to be difficult for you: it may be something that, if you had more assistance with it or just more of it, your parenting/caregiving would be easier. Don't share your word with others right now – we'll be doing this later." (After everyone has their hand up.) *"OK, what I'd like you to do right now is look around the group and, if you haven't already, notice the tremendous wealth of parental/caregiver resources we have here. You're going to pair up with someone you don't know well yet, but who looks like a person you might seek out for advice on parenting (not your spouse/partner).*

"After this is accomplished, we want you to be in your pairs and take five minutes to introduce yourselves, share a bit about yourself, and tell the

quality you thought of earlier and why you found it so important. Take 30 seconds to describe this word.

(Next)

"What we want you to do now is look at your partner and decide who is 'it' and who is 'not it.' I'd like all the 'its' to come with me and the 'not its' to go with Emery (other therapist). Before you go, make sure that you remember your partner's word as well as your own."

(After they reach the intended spot)

"We want you now to put on your blindfolds and let me place you around in different spots of the room, OK? Don't move or speak until I tell you to do so."

(After everyone has shared their words) *"Now try and find your partner using the following rules: (1) The only word you may speak is the quality you are searching for. For example, if the quality I shared is 'patience,' this is the only word I can speak when searching for my partner. I know it might be tempting, but you can't say, 'Hey, Bill, I'm over here.' You can (1) use the quality word to find your partner, (2) keep your eyes closed until you find your partner or feel unsafe and need to open them up, (3) when you find your partner, open your eyes and do a brief sort of congratulations, but then remain silent. If you understand these three rules, we want you to get into the "bumper" position we showed you earlier. If you have questions, raise one hand, and I will call on you. Is everyone ready? OK, begin."*

Debrief

These are some debriefing questions that may center the group.

- Were there any insights about parenting/caregiving that you will take with you to further consider or incorporate into your life at home?
- What was one of the things you found challenging in this activity? Does it relate in any way to challenges as a parent/caregiver?
- What conditions would need to change that could affect how you respond when parenting/caregiving?
- Have you considered or gained knowledge/skills using other resources (e.g., website, people, books) to support your parenting/ caregiving?
- Were you ever "stuck" in not knowing what to do in this activity? If so, what did you do and how was your manner to problem solve the same or different as a parent/caregiver?

Contraindications: If unable to use blindfold, then client can close eyes

#16. Path to recovery (Asking for help)

Therapeutic application

This activity can produce a high degree of confrontation. Before doing this activity, groups should:

1   Have worked together for a while
2   Have already established a sense of group identity
3   Feels relatively comfortable and safe when blindfolded.
4   Have previous adventure experiences involved with trust, support, and challenge issues.

When presented in this manner, this initiative emphasizes:

1   The ability of substance abusers to ask for help
2   Their ability to set appropriate boundaries around issues concerning their recovery and maintaining abstinence.
     For whom: Group: parents/caregivers
     Set-up and needs: Gentle, flat ground with 5–15 trees (or strong posts that support cord), 50 feet of cord, blindfolds for each person

Facilitation

The setup for this initiative uses some sort of cord/rope (e.g., strong cord) connected between five to 15 trees strung tightly at waist level in a chain (zigzag and straight for about 50 feet). The terrain where people walk is gentle since clients will be walking with blindfolds or closed eyes. Sharp, pointed branches on the tree trunks should also to be avoided. If the activity is conducted inside, chairs and other immovable objects can used in place of trees. Individuals are asked to wear blindfolds but are given the choice to do the initiative with their eyes closed if blindfolds are bothersome. After the clients are introduced to the initiative by a metaphoric description of the experience, they are led by the therapist to various points of the Maze. The participants have not seen the roped-off area of the Maze, and the usual precautions for physical safety are taken (e.g., no ducking under ropes, always maintain contact with one hand on the rope and the other hand out in front to keep from bumping into anyone).

All proper safety issues should be followed (e.g., making sure that there are no obstacles that people will run into or trip on, reinforcing that people should have one hand up in a "bumper" position, moving at a safe, slow speed while they are walking with their eyes closed). As a therapist, I make observations and address safety issues. As clients finish the activity, I encourage them to remain silent until everyone is finished.

Sample presentation

"The next activity is called the 'Path to recovery.' It's called that because several of the obstacles you'll encounter are very similar to obstacles many of you are currently facing in your addictions. Our addictions often define us in our path to a substance-free lifestyle, and we often fail because we don't remember to live by principles that will allow us to keep ourselves abstinent from abusive substances.

After you hear the directions, you will be placed on your road to recovery by putting your hand on the rope. This rope will lead you to a path of indeterminate length. Along your journey to recovery, you will meet various other people going in different directions. Some of these people will be in a great hurry, brimming with confidence. Others will be more tentative, moving cautiously. Some will seem to know the right way to go and the right direction, whereas others will seem lost. Don't let go of the rope, because if you do, you will lose the path, and I will have to ask you to stop until the activity ends.

The goal of your journey is to reach one of the exits of abstinence. There are several exits in this Maze, and as you reach one of these exits, I will be there to ask you two important questions: (1) Do you wish to step out of the Maze, or (2) Do you want to stay in the Maze? If you decide to step out of the Maze, I'll ask you to remove your blindfold and sit quietly in the abstinence area until this initiative is over. If you choose to go back into the Maze, you run the risk that this exit door may be shut when you return, and you will have to find another exit.

If, at any time during this activity, you would like to receive help, all you need to do is ask for it, and guidance will be given. Otherwise, we would like everyone to not speak throughout this initiative until it's completed. Remember the safety rules of the initiative we've provided and speak only if you want help. When you are at an exit, I'll be waiting for you and then will ask you to make your decisions. After approximately 30 minutes, I will ask those still in the Maze to open their eyes for a small break."

Participants are distributed throughout the Maze and instructed only to move once the go-ahead is given. When everyone has been placed in the Maze, participants are informed that they can begin to try to find an exit. In this initiative, however, the exit remains closed until a person asks for help. Asking for help is the key to opening the exit, and the person asking for help can decide to step out of the Maze to a place of sobriety or return to the Maze.

Some participants may still be in the Maze after the 30-minute limit is reached. This usually occurs because they keep returning to the Maze to rescue one another, even though each may have found an exit at least once. It's a judgment call on the therapist's part whether to keep permitting people to continually go back into the Maze or to ask them to join the abstinence group.

When the client arrive at an exit, they are quietly asked to decide. Therapist should do this without revealing the location of the exit to the other participants. If the participants choose to step out, they are quietly asked to remove their blindfolds or open their eyes and stand to the side to observe others in the Maze. It is important that these participants remain still and silent observers. If the participant chooses to return to the Maze, the exit closes, and the instructor should proceed with the initiative.

Debrief

Different issues come up with each group, but I usually begin the initiative by asking clients to relate their adventure experiences to their own experiences in trying to reach or maintain sobriety. A variety of issues come up, but the primary ones I tend to focus on are: (1) how does asking for help assist clients in this initiative; (2) client choices at the exits; and (3) what "failing to hold on" to the rope represented.

In the discussion, I make sure to inform clients that the exits weren't opened until someone asked for help and describe how asking for help directed this client to an exit. I also ask the client to elaborate on why they asked for help and what it felt like to receive assistance. The whole point of including this dynamic is to use a metaphor about the need for substance users to ask for help, particularly when feeling lost or "blinded" by their addiction.

Clients must place their recovery process first in any decision. Stepping out of the Maze represents a healthy personal decision. Choosing to go back in represents a dangerous decision, one where they may never be able to achieve an exit to abstinence again.

Some other important metaphors to include are:

- Letting go of the rope represents losing a chance to achieve abstinence.
- What were the feelings or observations of the people observing others lost in the maze of abusive substances?
- What were some metaphorical techniques participants used to find an exit to abstinence?
- How does the behavior of the client exhibited in this therapeutic experience match the behavior of where the client currently is in their recovery process?

#17. Play together – Stay together

Therapeutic application

The following case study is an example of using an adventure experience as a medium for change with a couple experiencing sexual intimacy issues. In working with this couple, I used the framework of the activity "Boundary Setting" with "Push off/Take a Step/Collaborative Competition" with several extensions/variations to mirror the clients' issues and potential resolutions.

The objective of this adventure experience was to assist this couple in rewriting their "script" for sexual intimacy. This couple included a client who identified as a male (John) and a client who identified as a female (Martha). They had been married for 13 years and had two sons together. Martha had been a victim of sexual abuse as a young girl. This experience had overshadowed their ability to be sexually intimate with one another throughout their relationship, but at this time, it seemed to be problematic. As John would engage and initiate sexual intimacy, she would experience flashbacks and dissociative states that were difficult and troublesome. The power and prevalence of these experiences were also beginning to affect other areas of their relationship. While I saw all family members during several sessions, at this time, just John and Martha attended the therapy session.

For whom: Partners: adult couples

Set-up and needs: Open space of about 25 feet, rolling chairs (optional if standing for a long period of time is a contraindication)

Facilitation

This activity takes one to three sessions. During the first session, the couple will be asked to do a "walking" activity that invites one client to ask permission to walk closer to the other client after being given approval. For this reason, the therapist needs to decide who will be the "walker" and who will be the "permission giver." The couple stands 25 feet apart and the "walker" asks if they can take a few steps toward the other person. Before moving, the "permission giver" needs to respond with "You can come closer" or "I want you to stay where you are." This request and response continues until the "permission giver" says "I want you to stay where you are" (the "walker" stops). The couple remains in their respective positions to let their feelings resonate (the therapist can consider giving cues to close eyes, etc.). The couple is then invited to talk about how they feel at this moment. The therapist then invites the couple to sit down and discuss other therapeutic goals. The therapist needs to decide if they want to give homework to the couple, which could include no sex for the following week. This is the end of session one.

For session two, the couple begins again at 25 feet apart in the same roles as session one. The "walker" asks permission to move closer and the "permission giver" says "You can come closer" or "I want you to stay where you are." If the response is "I want you to stay where you are," the "walker" asks "Can you tell me what you need?" The therapist supports the couple in a dialogue while standing. The therapist then invites the couple to sit down and discuss other therapeutic goals. The therapist needs to decide if they want to give homework to the couple which could include no sex for the following week again. This is the end of session two.

For session three, the couple returns to the same 25 feet starting points and does the same activity with the same question and response. If the couple gets to the point where they are standing close enough that they could touch hands, the therapist invites them to put their hands in front of them, palm to palm without touching. The "permission giver" can then choose to keep their eyes open and slowly move their hands. At the same time, the "walker" is invited to close their eyes and follow the warmth of the hands of the "permission giver's." If having eyes closed doesn't work for the "walker" they can keep their eyes open. The therapist supports the couple in a dialogue while standing. The therapist then invites the couple to sit down and discuss other therapeutic goals. Depending upon the degree of comfort regarding their intimacy and feelings, the couple determines whether they are ready for increased intimacy.

Sample presentation

"I'd like to do an exercise with the two of you to have you explore what may be currently happening in your relationship. While facing one another from across the room, I invite you both to stand with your palms up at your side. John will walk toward Martha. In this process, Martha will direct John as to how close to her he can walk. Martha, the guideline for you to use is that John can walk toward you only as long as you feel comfortable. At the first sign that you feel uncomfortable to the point where you do not feel you can handle your "uncomfortableness," you need to tell John to stop, and he must stop. In fact, ask him to back up to a point where you feel comfortable with his distance from you. (We did this exercise several times until John and Martha could stand together with their palms barely touching.)

Now that you have arrived in this comfortable position, I want you to work together to try "cooperative touching." Standing toe to toe and palm to palm as you are, I would like John to try to follow Martha's movements in slow motion. Martha guides you, and John, you do your best to follow her lead. There may be times when you can pick up Martha's cues and guidance, John. There may also be other times when John may have diffi-culty following Martha's cues and guidance. While both scenarios may exist, I encourage the two of you to explore what works when John can follow Martha and what to do differently when John cannot follow Martha's guidance. I encourage the two of you to explore the different positions you can guide one another to without feeling uncomfortable and enjoying the presence and love of one another."

Debrief

The experience was debriefed with the therapist, focusing on how the couple's relationship needs to start with Martha initially guiding John in areas where she felt comfortable. Once that began to be established, I told the couple that there probably would come a time when Martha could feel comfortable in having John guide her. This experience was pivotal in rewriting the couple's script around being intimate with one another and extended toward other aspects of the relationship.

Contraindications: If clients are unable to stand for an extended period of time, they can use rolling chairs. Also, if there exists a situation of abuse, accommodations need to be made to ensure the safety of both clients. Introducing an experience with this much confrontation to unprepared clients would contraindicate treatment. It is also important to leave a great deal of time for processing individuals with group issues before and after the experience

#18. Scarf pull

Therapeutic application

This activity is one of my favorites when a person's partner doesn't come to couples therapy. This kinesthetic metaphor quickly draws a client's attention to conscious and unconscious attributes of an identified relationship (e.g., the "push and pull" with relationships and follower/leader issues with couples). This activity can work well when the therapeutic goal is to examine the relationship between couples.

For whom: Individuals: parents/caregivers

Set-up and needs: One scarf, other "scarf-like" items that can be pulled by two people

Facilitation

This therapist invites the client to hold onto one end of the scarf. When this happens, the therapist begins by giving a gentle tug on the scarf and adds increasingly stronger "tugs" until the client must let go or begins to tug back. As the therapist adds stronger tugs, the client typically will demonstrate (project) their relationship structure onto the experience (e.g., if the client lets go soon it could represent "giving in," if the client pulls back with equal force, it could represent an equivalent investment during conflicts). As a therapist, you are trying to mirror the client's attachment between two people.

Debrief

As part of the reflection process, you address the areas where your words connect with the actions that occur in the activity. For example, you may say, "How is your relationship with this person?" and they will share that meaning with you. At the same time, you mirror activities with their words. For example, when you talk about the tug of relationships or the give and take in relationships, you pull on the rope to connect the two realities together. Your dialogue introduces the activity and its meaning for the client.

Variations: if a person does not have a scarf, you can use a tie. But please note that a tie/belt may represent a entirely different type of reality/ connotation or prescription.

#19. Stepping stones (Field of problems)

Therapeutic application

This activity could help treat clients struggling with impulse control and needing proactive problem-solving skills. Clients with substance use issues might also benefit, especially if a conversation about maintenance and relapse is engaged. Growth may also be made with couples who are struggling to solve problems.

This activity illustrates how everyone's path is filled with potential obstacles. The key to navigating life effectively is to learn how to anticipate and avoid obstacles while dealing with them proactively when they are encountered. The activity should be framed to the client's specific problem-solving needs, whether the client makes it across or continues to beat their previous distance records.

For whom: Group of 4–20 put into partners: adults, adolescents

Set-up and needs: Open space and obstacles on the ground that could represent substance use

Facilitation

You can design a course out of available objects that are the "problem" obstacles. If you are inside an office, you can use chairs and tables or other objects that can be bumped into gently and not break. If you are outside, things like trees and bushes or other natural landscape elements can be used. Use notebooks, water bottles, or any other loose objects inside that will be felt by the client if they bump into them. It is important that the participant does not see the course ahead of time; it is also more fun. This activity typically involves blindfolding the participant (if not contra-indicated), as the goal is to move from one end of the obstacle course to the other without meeting an obstacle. The facilitator's or assigned part-ner's job is to guide the client verbally. Typically, the client is walking away from the voice guiding them. The rules for bumping into an obstacle should be framed to the life scenario a client is currently dealing with. Clear penalties can be co-created by the client and facilitator after the first try. This usually helps clients take ownership of the activity. Some sug-gestions for consequences could be a delay of five seconds, a re-start, or a question about problem-solving in the client's real life. If the client answers the question innovatively and realistically, they can restart from that point.

Debrief

The participant should be careful in choosing their guide or voice in this activity. Discussing what they look for in a guiding force to maneuver them through the obstacle course could be an interesting way to look at this activity. Another way to debrief would be to have the participant identify the obstacles in their life and name each before they start. They could also choose to name who their guides are in the outside world.

Contraindications: Anyone made uncomfortable wearing blindfolds

#20. The system

Therapeutic application

The purpose of this therapeutic experience has been primarily to address sys-tems issues of a social organization. The application presented here is one for a family, but certainly, any group looking at ways to see themselves as more than just individual parts or members is a possible application for this experience.

I have used this activity with families in "traditional family therapy rooms" and outdoor settings. I use the learning experience to provide insight into how family members interact with one another. You'll also gain a pretty good idea of how "playful" family members are and the level of their enjoyment in being with one another, as well as how well they can interpret learning from experiential approaches to therapy.

The experience tends to provide information on:

- The systemic interaction of a family,
- How family members interact with one another, as well as a "struc-tural" picture of family alliances, rules, and enmeshed and disengaged family behavior, and
- The potential of family members to interpret learnings from experi-ential therapy approaches.

For whom: Group: couples, families

Set-up and needs: Each group needs a paper cup, bandana, water source or small dry beans if water is not appropriate

Facilitation

One of the wonderful features of this activity is the minimal and accessible nature of the props. You only need a regular-size bandana or cloth napkin, an unbreakable cup (e.g., non-leaking paper, plastic), and a substance to fill the cup (e.g., water, sand, uncooked rice).

Ask the family to spread the napkin/bandana on a flat surface like a large table or floor. Place the cup in the center of the bandana. Have them fill up the cup with water or another substance to the level of challenge they desire. Note that inverted-shaped cups are more challenging than straight-sided cups.

After this is done, I ask the family to grab the edges of the bandana with both hands and not let go until they reach the end of their task. The bandana must be held taut, and they cannot come in physical contact with the cup. As a group, they must travel with the bandana and cup from where they are to their destination without spilling the cup.

Sample presentation

(Presentation started in a circle where each family member can see one another and the therapist) *"After listening to you talk about issues you face, I was struck by how each of you contributes to and worries about your family. Both as individual members and as a family, you are concerned in one way or another about meeting your needs. I am somewhat curious if, with all of these 'parts,' there possibly is a bit more that exists within your family.*

I want to invite you to do an activity with me that might give us a clue as to what some of those 'parts' are. Besides having a bit of fun during the activity, have your 'antenna up' to see what these might be. Okay? Let's give it a go then."

Depending on the family, I make the path I ask them to travel as difficult (as well as metaphoric) as needed. Additional challenges such as going over or under objects, up and down stairs, or squeezing through narrow passages/doors can "up the ante" of the challenge.

(Remember that water may spill. Be sure the room you are in can accommodate this "outcome." Dried beans or other small objects can be a substitute for places where water cannot be used.)

One great additional element to the learning experience is asking each family member to trace their hand onto the bandana and write on each finger a quality of importance (e.g., something you stand for, something you value in the family, what you like to do for fun in the family, how the family lets you know you're important/valuable/loved, the most important thing you think the family needs to work on).

Debrief

There are a variety of debriefing models one can follow, but I center most of my attention on:

- What happened?
- What were the consequences of what happened?
- How does what happened relate to what is going on with the family at an interactive level? For example, observing how the family handles success and failure as a group can provide valuable assessment and insight.

I also focus on the solutions rather than the problems associated with the family system processes. Examples of this type of perspective include:

- Center on enhancing the solution rather than the problem
- Look at what the clients are doing right rather than what clients are doing wrong
- Emphasize what clients want rather than what clients don't want
- Seek to accentuate positive client strengths rather than eliminate negative client weaknesses
- Be interested in when the problem doesn't happen rather than "why" the problem occurs (e.g., look for exceptions to the problem rather than what "causes" and "maintains" the problem)

#21. Turning over a new leaf

Therapeutic application

This activity involves possible involvement in problem-solving, creativity, communication, and leadership tasks. "Turning over a new leaf" is an expression often associated with this activity, especially when creating a group vision, change in direction, or new beginning.

For whom: Groups: unlimited numbers; adults, adolescents

Set-up and needs: One large tarp, blanket, or tablecloth to serve as the "leaf," light colored duct tape or wide masking tape, several permanent markers

Facilitation

The activity begins with a tarp laid flat on the floor/ground and all participants standing on one side. The goal is for the group to finish all standing on the other side of the tarp without touching the floor/ground or coming off the tarp. The entire tarp must flip over.

One side of the tarp is designated as the top side, or the "present" time frame, and the underside of the tarp represents the "future" time frame. The floor/ground represents the past.

Ask each client to write short descriptions (1–3 words) on a strip of duct/masking tape about a behavior they would like to change. Examples might be poor communication, doing the same old thing, being afraid to make mistakes, or experiencing too many changes too fast. Tape these comments randomly on the top (present) side of the tarp.

When all are finished, ask if anyone would like to share what they wrote about their present experience, Then ask clients to identify what behaviors they could do instead. Ask them to answer the following questions: What would you do to nurture these behaviors? What would you need, wish, desire, etc.? Encourage the group to keep responses focused and relevant.

Now, ask all clients to stand on the "leaf" (the tarp). Their task is to turn the tarp over without touching the floor or stepping off it. Strategizing begins as the group stands together on the tarp. Tarp size is critical to the challenge level: the larger the tarp, the easier the challenge. Experiment with the tarp size before you offer the initiative. About two square feet per person is a good rule of thumb. If the group accomplishes the turn easily, challenge them to fold the tarp smaller and smaller!

Turn the tarp back to the "present side" and invite clients to consider any descriptions of the future that they would like to shift to the Variation: Put all tapes on a board and begin to create the common group vision.

Debrief

- What are the factors that can affect changes in your life?
- What are the factors that you need to consider when making decisions?
- How do you deal with difficult past events?
- How do you handle change? When did things go better than other times?
- What happened or didn't happen when this took place?

#22. Warp speed (Group juggle)

Therapeutic application

The activity is generally used to help improve communication, follow established boundaries (tossing pattern), and build teamwork. It can also be used for assessment and to indicate possible treatment interventions. This activity requires cooperation and teamwork so depending upon the clients, conflicts may arise and they may take on different roles when in a group setting.

For who: Groups: 5–15 adults, adolescents

Set-up and needs: To prepare for this activity, you will need 3-5 (or more!) objects that can be tossed and caught easily. These things can be as simple as a scrunched up piece of paper.

Facilitation

Clear an area so the participants can stand in a circle. Ask them to raise one hand and explain that a raised hand means they have not caught and tossed an object. To establish the tossing pattern for this activity, call someone's name and toss underhand (when tossing arm is straight and hand is beside leg) an object to them. Cue clients to remember who they received the ball from and tossed it to. This person continues to say a person's name and toss the object. After you catch and toss keep your hand down. Continue until everyone has received and thrown. Check in with clients to confirm they know who they caught from and tossed to. Redo toss pattern if necessary.

Now that the ball tossing pattern is set. You can use any "gimmick" to pick a client to begin with the ball (e.g., who has the next birthday, lowest number home address number) and give this person the object. Tell the clients that this is a timed activity. They must send the object to the same person they threw it to before. The object must begin with the person who starts it. Give them a countdown to begin (Ready, 3, 2, 1, Go!). This round will be the group's baseline time. Share with the group and invite them to try and get faster.

Now, reiterate the rules: the item must touch everyone in the same order, and it must begin and end with the same person. Ask them if they are ready to go but if they say they want some time to plan/strategize then that is fine. Continue trying the activity multiple times and share the time. It may be therapeutically appropriate to challenge the group to a faster time by reiterating the rules (i.e., the rule doesn't say the object needs to be tossed but only touched).

Debrief

To reflect on this activity, you might discuss the group goals and the decisions made throughout this activity. Additionally, you might discuss the communication and feelings that arose throughout the activity. A few example questions for reflection include:

1 How did you make decisions throughout this activity? Were you willing to adapt your solution based on the previous attempt?
2 What role did you play in the activity? Leader? Follower? Quiet? Loud?

Variations

There are many ways to modify this activity. A few ideas include:

1 Have an object move in both directions (e.g., regular pattern and in reverse order) at the same time

2   Use an object that is harder to catch
3   Add more objects to catch and toss
4   Ask clients to think up another way to complete this activity

#23. Wrestling with conflict (Thumb/Arm wrestling)

Therapeutic application

Many individuals, couples, and groups sometimes find themselves in conflict due to the social paradigms and mental models they possess. Such belief systems often direct their thoughts and actions toward negative interdependencies and unintended consequences. One such situation is when one person feels the need to "get ahead" at the expense of others (e.g., "I win, you lose"). In response, this can lead to the individuals trying to "one-up" their partners in return. This often results in a escalating pattern where the focus is for ME to win and you to lose verses both of us winning.

Breaking out of these belief systems often requires a different thinking pattern (e.g., "thinking outside of the box"). This experiential activity can accomplish this by placing participants in a traditional paradigm while rewarding actions and thought processes that transcend conflictual or dysfunctional behavior.

There are many variations for this activity for it to be tailored around the needs of the clients. Some therapists have adapted this activity in the following ways:

1   Couples in conflict, particularly those with a long history of failed efforts to resolve power struggles.
2   Peer groups in conflict with one another.
3   Parents/caregivers and adolescent children who conflict with one another

For whom: Partners/couples: adults, adolescents
Set-up and needs: Flat surface for partners (on floor/ground or table-tops), small wrapped candies or small objects to use for counting points (optional)

Facilitation

Choose arm-wrestling or thumb wrestling as the selected activity. Arm wrestling can present a more vivid representation of the learning experience, but the group or surroundings may dictate what you choose (i.e., the group may not be able to handle the emotional directness of arm wrestling, the physical structure of the room may not allow it to take place).

I begin the experience by inviting the group to pair up with an individual with the same size bicep muscle as them. In making this request, I often get a quizzical look or two in response to my statement. So, I repeat my request, often rolling up the sleeves of my shirt and pointing to my bicep muscle. As people pair up, I state that some group members may have done this activity before. Borrowing a partner or using a co-therapist, I demonstrate the starting position of arm wrestling, where people clasp hands. I inform the group that each time an individual can pin down their partner's hand to the ground, they will receive one point and are to return to the starting position of the activity and begin again. I informed the group that they will be given 15 seconds to acquire as many points as possible. If I have M&M candies with me, I tell them I will distribute candy after the activity, with one candy for each point they acquire. I ask if there are any questions and quickly ask participants to get in position so I may begin the 15 seconds.

After I say "go," I inform the participants when five seconds and ten seconds have passed and ask them to stop when the 15 seconds are completed. I invite those people who were able to earn at least one point to raise their hand, then those able to earn at least three points to raise their hand, followed by people able to earn at least five points or more to raise their hand. Then, I go around the room and distribute M&Ms to each participant. These two methods used together tend to punctuate differences between individual scores.

Many individuals in the group do not receive a point and most individuals receive two points at most. If no one has received more than five points, I conduct the experience again, reiterating the rules of the activity. However, after performing the experience for a couple of rounds, one or more participants will acquire 20 or more points. This becomes more surprising when both individuals in the paired relationship achieve a relatively astounding number of points/candies. Such a radical difference in scores across the group can produce great interest in how an individual acquired so many points or sometimes comments like "they must've cheated."

Once a solution is found (e.g., a method producing a win-win paradigm instead of a win-lose paradigm), groups move quickly to implement a nontraditional strategy to this activity. I often will have one of the pairs of individuals accumulating many points demonstrate their strategy to the rest of the group.

Debrief

While the learning can be self-evident from the experience, reflective dialogue can present valuable shared learning experiences and punctuate connections for clients. One debriefing model uses the questions, "What?

So what? Now what?" It is an easy and flexible manner for strengthening the learning from the experience. Other direct questions to utilize for appropriate groups include:

- What happened?
- Were there things that kept you from being more productive?
- What led you to opportunities to see possibilities of more productive/functional behavior?
- Do you see similar patterns of behavior in your current life?
- What will you do in the future that will encourage you to see and implement such behavior possibilities?

Contraindications

This can be a very powerful exercise for groups, particularly ones in conflictual relationships or highly competitive. The activity sometimes triggers presenting issues. Thumb wrestling would be more appropriate for such individuals. People who are unable to eat chocolate can select another kind of reward.

#24. Your cup has holes!

Therapeutic approach

Sometimes, therapeutic issues draw so much energy and resources away from the client they become unable to move to resolve anything. It's as if any energy reservoir they have is being drained away. This draining must be addressed before progress can resolve any of their issues. The following activity will help provide a visual and tactile example of how this works and hopefully begin a discussion of what must be done for that individual to "raise the level" of their energy reservoir.

Some populations that might benefit from insight from the activity could be:

- Clients dealing with substance abuse issues (specifically discussing how using feeds the "drains").
- Clients suffering from anxiety and/or depression.
- Clients recovering from breakdowns who are beginning to re-engage with the complexity of life again.

For whom: Groups, pairs/couples, individuals: adults, older school-age children

Set-up and needs: A paper cup, sharp pencil, permanent marker, water source, or dry small beans (optional) for each person. A tray or dishpan to "catch" water/beans (optional)

Facilitation

Begin by asking the client to choose one goal that the cup represents. Perhaps it's as simple as having more energy to complete the basic tasks necessary for life. Perhaps it's a goal that will require a much higher level of functioning. Whatever the client chooses, ask them to draw a line on the cup where they think the reservoir of their energy is and where they believe it will need to be for them to start moving forward. Then, ask clients to recall things that have been draining their energy lately. As they name these items have clients poke holes in the cup, putting the most draining things to the bottom. The more manageable items toward the top. This begins to create a visual and tactile metaphor for their situation. Pouring water/beans into the cup may be unnecessary, but seeing whether they would put the holes in the same places when water is poured in (and begins to pour out!) might be more powerful.

Debrief

This activity can begin a discussion about how clients want to approach the "drains" in their lives and in what order of priority. It is important for the therapist to ask about the placement of specific holes that the visual and physical representation illustrates. The overwhelm accompanying such a "draining" experience can be addressed by working on one hole at a time, perhaps discussing how that hole could be moved farther up the side of the cup. One minor adjustment to one hole may affect others, but the debrief is the time to work with the client to envision getting to a place that is a bit less draining. This is facilitated by brainstorming ways to adjust the level of the holes, along with how to shrink or plug them up. The discussion may lead to talking about having other people help by putting a finger over one of the holes. Discussion may ensue around how quickly many other people can get dragged into helping when short-term solutions are the only ones practiced. One goal of this activity is to apply a strengths-based and solution-focused lens. A possible progression of questioning, following Bloom's taxonomy of transfer of learning, might include:

- How did you decide where to place each "drain" hole?
- What are the top three "drains" for you?
- Are any of these "drains" like each other? If so, what do they have in common?
- What do you see as the leading cause of these "drains"?
- What has worked to "plug the drain" in the past?
- What about the placement of these "drains"? What might it look like if you re-ordered their placement?
- What would you do to "move" a drain a little higher up the cup wall?

- How would this affect the other "drains"?
- What would you notice about your "cup" if just one drain were moved or removed? (Address each drain separately if necessary and in terms relevant to its nature.)
- How can you move/remove this drain from what we've just discussed?

Contraindications

If a participant is in a pre-contemplative stage, engaging them in more action-oriented discussion may be best.

11 Digital access to adventure therapy activities and techniques: Kikori

Kendra Bostick

Digital access to information about adventure therapy could be an asset for the adventure therapist. Professionals will benefit from the ease of accessing a digital resource that includes the opportunity to collaborate with other therapists. One resource that provides adventure therapists access to thousands of experiential activities is Kikori. This digital platform supports therapists and educators in helping youth develop social emotional learning (SEL) skills. This aids facilitators in traditional office, school, and outdoor settings and is designed to be a valuable addition to a therapist's toolkit.

This chapter provides an overview of how a digital platform like Kikori can be used to match therapeutic activities to clients' specific needs. By doing so, practitioners can discover activities and curriculum that align with therapeutic outcomes. To access a free trial of Kikori, follow these steps.

1   Go to: https://www.kikoriapp.com.
2   Sign up using your email and password.
3   Discover activities and playlists to use within your therapeutic practice.

The importance of access to effective treatment strategies

Substance use during adolescence lies at the very confluence of worsening trends in mental health care (NSDUH, 2019). Adolescence is associated with multiple processes that compound a client's vulnerability, including, but not limited to, identity formation, greater responsibilities, the influence of peer relations in decision-making, and the emergence of more complex thinking. Developmental factors underpinning impulsivity also contribute to the negative synergistic relationship between substance use disorder (SUD) and mental health problems (SAMHSA, 2020). Mental, emotional, and behavioral disorders among youth cost the nation $247 billion yearly due to crime, health services, and lost productivity (Eisenberg & Neighbors, 2007). Although youth are not necessarily involved in the labor market, their disorders can impact families and other related systems in ways that have rippling economic costs – and costs that do not readily translate to dollars and

DOI: 10.4324/9781032640303-11

cents. Many of these costly disorders begin to present early in life, suggesting efforts to prevent them should be addressed during adolescence.

In the ever-evolving landscape of adventure therapy, the integration of digital access has emerged as a transformative tool for therapists seeking effective and engaging activities. The dynamic nature of digital platforms offers unparalleled personalization, allowing therapists to tailor activities to individual needs and preferences. Moreover, these platforms facilitate communication among therapists through technological features, fostering collaboration and the exchange of innovative ideas. The omnipresent accessibility of digital resources, available at one's fingertips wherever they may be, breaks down geographical barriers and ensures that adventure therapy is not confined to a specific location. The shift from traditional methods, like pulling out a book, to interactive apps further enhances the therapeutic experience, particularly with teenagers. The ability to choose between activities on an app fosters a sense of autonomy and choice, potentially increasing their buy-in and engagement in the therapeutic process.

Kikori: Digital access to adventure therapy at your fingertips

Kikori is a community-driven platform that provides therapists with easy access to thousands of therapeutic activities involving active play and intentional reflection. Its value lies in the versatility and depth of engaging activities that can be accessed anywhere by the touch of a screen. Kikori utilizes an experiential Social Emotional Learning (eSEL) approach that offers behavioral health practitioners the tools needed to help their clients cultivate connections, community, and a sense of belonging. New and seasoned therapists can access activities that are divided into categories aligned with group development standards (e.g., ice melters, energizers, team builders, and problem solvers) as well as those aligned with CASEL (Collaborative Academic Social and Emotional Learning Standards) (self-awareness, self-management, social awareness, relationship skills and responsible decision-making). Kikori activities can also be filtered for different ages, group structure, materials available, energy level (sitting, moving and running activities), and type of activity (e.g., check-ins, assessments, focus games, appreciations, etc.), and are available online, via tablet or mobile devices, allowing easy anytime access to activities and reflection questions. All activities can also be shared with colleagues and printed in PDF format.

How Kikori's eSEL approach works

Experiential Social Emotional Learning (eSEL), exemplified by Kikori, integrates active play and intentional reflection for youth to acquire, practice, and apply Social Emotional Learning (SEL) skills, drawing on Kolb's experiential learning cycle (Donnellan & Jack, 2014). Kikori's activities aim to foster connections, community, and a sense of belonging, providing mental health clinicians with tools to create an inviting space for youth growth. Grounded in experiential education, Kikori emphasizes reflection as vital for group development and SEL. Following a research-based experiential learning model, Kikori's Play, Reflect, Connect, Grow process ensures purposeful play aligns with intentional reflection, facilitating meaningful learning and the development of intra- and interpersonal connections in a supportive community environment.

Through play and reflection, therapists have the unique opportunity to reach ALL areas of the brain! According to one of the top researchers in experiential education and neuroscience, knowledge resides in a network of neurons in the neocortex (Zull, 2011). Learning from experience results in modification, growth, and pruning of these neurons, synapses, and neural networks. Learning physically changes the brain and educating is the art of changing the brain (Zull, 2011). When youth play a new activity, instead of linear learning, they have a spiral of learning where they assimilate the new knowledge into what they already know! Figure 11.1 shows how youth move through the Play-Reflect-Connect-Grow process and that areas in the brain are engaged:

- Play provides concrete information from the outside world that begins the cycle in the sensory cortex area of the brain.
- Reflect provides time to create meaningful observations by asking clients "what happened" during the activity in the back integrative cortex of the brain.
- Connect occurs in the frontal integrative cortex and helps us think and problem solve using "so what" questions.
- Grow facilitates action when asked "now what" during an experience in the motor cortex of the brain.

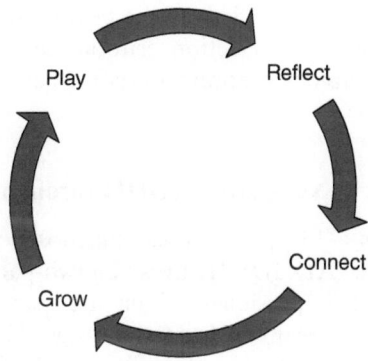

Figure 11.1 The Play-Reflect-Connect-Grow process

How to use Kikori with clients

Kikori provides therapists with the ability to easily search for activities specific to their population, resources available and outcomes sought after.

1   Sign up at www.kikoriapp.com and create your unique login.
2   Discover adventure therapy activities that build social emotional skills aligned with treatment outcomes.
3   Utilize activities during sessions with clients.
4   Log notes to track which skills clients are developing and mastering.

There are several important factors that you should take into consideration when planning activities and using the platform's filter (Bostick and Lottig, 2022).

1   Age of your client(s): How old is your client and what developmental stage are they at?
2   Time commitment: How much time do you have available to lead the activity?
3   Energy level: What energy level is appropriate for this activity? Do you want your clients to be sitting (low energy), moving (middle energy), or running (high energy)?
4   Materials available: What materials are available to use with your clients?
5   Outcomes: What are your treatment goals? What outcomes are you working toward?

This section presents fictional case study presentations of three types of clients (individual youth, family, and young adult), providing the client background, challenges being faced by that particular client, potential assessment tools, review of the client's strengths and interest, adventure therapy activity selection criteria, selected activities (available in Kikori), implementation, outcome and future steps, and conclusion.

Case study 1: Alex – Navigating ADHD through team building

Background: Alex is a 13-year-old male, diagnosed with attention deficit hyperactivity disorder (ADHD). He lives in a two-parent household with a younger sibling. Alex is passionate about art, particularly drawing and painting, and exhibits creativity beyond his age. He faces challenges in maintaining focus in school, struggles with impulsivity, and often experiences difficulty in regulating emotions which impacts his relationships with peers.

Challenges:

1 Academic struggles: Alex's ADHD affects his academic performance due to difficulties in sustaining attention during lectures and completing assignments on time.
2 Impulsivity: Alex tends to act on impulses without considering consequences, leading to occasional conflicts with peers and authority figures.
3 Emotional regulation: Managing frustration and anger is a consistent challenge for Alex, affecting his social interactions.

Assessment:

• Utilized standardized ADHD assessments to identify specific areas of difficulty.
• Conducted interviews with Alex, parents, and teachers to gather comprehensive information about his behavior in various settings.
• Observed Alex's artistic abilities and the calming effect art has on him.

Strengths and Interests:

• Creativity: Alex has a strong passion for art, which serves as an outlet for self-expression.
• Social Interest: Despite occasional challenges, Alex expresses a desire for positive social interactions and values friendships.
• Kinesthetic learner: Alex learns best through hands-on experiences and activities.

Interventions: The therapist aims to address self-regulation challenges through team building activities that align with Alex's strengths and interests.

Adventure Therapy Activity Selection Criteria:

1 Artistic expression: Given Alex's passion for art, activities involving collaborative art projects could be beneficial for enhancing focus and self-regulation. *Select Kikori Attribute:* Creative Game
2 Structured challenges: Designing activities with clear instructions and goals to help Alex practice sustained attention and decision-making. *Select SEL Standard:* Impulse Control
3 Social integration: Incorporating activities that encourage positive social interactions to foster friendships and improve emotional regulation. *Select SEL Standard:* Social Engagement

Selected Kikori Adventure Therapy Activities:

1   Compliment the masterpiece: Engage Alex in a group project where each participant contributes to a larger mural. This activity promotes teamwork, patience, and sustained focus on a shared goal.
2   Helium loop: A structured group team building activity can provide a challenging yet controlled environment for Alex to practice problem-solving and decision-making skills
3   Paper drop: Incorporate social activities for Alex to practice focusing and self-regulation within a game context as well as building interpersonal skills.

Implementation:

- The therapist introduces each activity gradually, ensuring clear instructions and providing ample support.
- Regular debriefing sessions allow Alex to reflect on the experience and discuss challenges and successes.

Outcome and Future Steps:

- Initial observations show improvements in Alex's ability to focus, make decisions, and regulate emotions during team building activities.
- Future steps involve reinforcing these skills in different contexts, collaborating with teachers, and exploring additional tailored interventions.

Conclusion: Alex's journey showcases the importance of leveraging a youth client's strengths and interests in therapeutic interventions. Team building activities tailored to individual needs can significantly contribute to the development of self-regulation skills in the context of ADHD.

Case study 2: The Thompson family – Nurturing communication and connection

Background: The Thompson family consists of parents, Maria and Tyrone, and their two teenage children, Keisha (16) and Jalen (14). The family sought therapy due to escalating communication issues, leading to frequent misunderstandings and conflicts. Maria and Tyrone work full-time, often leaving little time for family bonding. Keisha is academically driven, while Jalen struggles with feelings of being overlooked.

Challenges:

1   Communication breakdown: The family experiences difficulty expressing emotions and needs, leading to frequent misunderstandings.

2   Time constraints: Maria and Tyrone's busy work schedules limit quality family time, impacting communication and connection.
3   Sibling dynamics: Keisha's academic focus sometimes overshadows Jalen's needs, contributing to his feelings of being overlooked.

Assessment:

• Conducted family interviews to understand each member's perspective on communication challenges.
• Utilized family genogram and communication assessments to identify patterns and areas for improvement.
• Explored individual interests and hobbies of each family member.

Strengths and Interests:

• Shared love for nature: The family enjoys spending time outdoors and has expressed a shared interest in hiking and camping.
• Individual hobbies: Keisha is passionate about photography, while Jalen enjoys playing musical instruments.
• Desire for connection: Despite the challenges, all family members express a longing for improved communication and stronger connections.

Interventions: The therapist aims to address communication issues through team-building activities that align with the family's strengths and interests.
Selected Kikori Adventure Therapy Activities:

1   Family sculpting: Given the family's need to improve communication, this activity provides family members with the opportunity to identify and work through dynamics that occur within their family as well as express their individual interests.
2   Finding solutions: Engaging in activities that require cooperation and teamwork to foster mutual understanding and support.
3   The system: Incorporating activities that provide a challenge will allow families to see how their interactions affect their family goals, providing them an opportunity to reflect on how they treat one another.

Any of these activities can be a precursor to inviting the family to take part in a family camping trip for 1–2 days, where they can put into practice some of the new actions they seek to bring into their family unit.
Implementation:

• The therapist introduces each activity gradually, ensuring clear expectations and providing guidance.

- Reflection sessions are incorporated to discuss each family member's experience and insights gained from the activities.

Outcome and Future Steps:

- Initial observations indicate improved communication and connection during team-building activities.
- The therapist works with the family to translate these positive experiences into everyday communication, reinforcing new patterns and habits.

Conclusion: The Thompson family's journey illustrates the power of tailored team-building activities to address communication issues. By aligning interventions with the family's strengths and interests, the therapist can facilitate meaningful connections and promote self-regulation skills within the family dynamic.

Case study 3: Mariana – Building a path to wellness

Background: Mariana is a 22-year-old college student who has sought therapy due to struggles with substance use, particularly alcohol. Mariana reports using alcohol as a way to cope with stress and anxiety related to academic pressures and social interactions. The substance use has started affecting academic performance and personal relationships.
   Challenges:

1   Substance use as coping mechanism: Mariana relies on alcohol to manage stress and anxiety, leading to unhealthy coping mechanisms.
2   Academic pressures: High academic expectations contribute to feelings of inadequacy and the need to escape through substance use.
3   Isolation: Mariana has started withdrawing from social activities, leading to a sense of loneliness and a lack of healthy connections.

Assessment:

- Conducted a substance use assessment to understand the extent of the issue and identify triggers.
- Explored Mariana's academic and personal life stressors contributing to substance use.
- Assessed Mariana's interests, hobbies, and social support networks.

Strengths and Interests:

- Seeking improved relationships: Mariana has a keen interest in building more interpersonal relationships with other college students.
- Love for nature: Enjoys spending time outdoors, especially in natural settings.

- Desire for change: Mariana acknowledges the need for a healthier life-style and expresses a desire to connect with others in a meaningful way.

Interventions: The therapist aims to address substance use issues and promote happiness and health through team-building activities that align with Mariana's strengths and interests.
  Adventure Therapy Activity Selection Criteria:

1 Interactive activities: Providing Mariana with an opportunity to work together with others while promoting self-discovery, stress relief, and emotional regulation.
2 Nature-based activities: Incorporating outdoor activities to leverage Mariana's love for nature, fostering a sense of well-being and connection.
3 Social connection: Choosing activities that encourage positive social interactions and help rebuild a supportive network.

Selected Adventure Therapy Activities:

1 Path to recovery (Asking for help): Facilitate this activity to provide an opportunity to learn Mariana's natural inclination to asking for help and how to begin requesting support from others.
2 Handling what you've got (Homeostasis): Introduce an activity that helps Mariana learn how she can maintain balance in her life through self-regulation and determination.
3 Embracing change: Utilize a simple exercise that Mariana can employ anywhere she goes that involves mindfulness and self-awareness.

Any of the activities above could be led in nature and may be combined with local AA programs.
  Implementation:

- The therapist introduces each activity with a focus on its potential benefits for stress reduction and well-being.
- Group discussions and reflection sessions are incorporated to process emotions and experiences during and after each activity.

Outcome and Future Steps:

- Initial observations indicate a positive impact on Mariana's mood, reduced substance use, and increased engagement in healthier activities.
- The therapist works with Mariana to translate the skills learned in team-building activities into daily life, reinforcing positive habits and coping mechanisms.

Appendix: Ethical guidelines for certified adventure therapists

Association for experiential education

Statement of purpose

Since adventure therapy profoundly affects individual lives, it is the purpose of these guidelines to advocate for the education, empowerment, and safety of those who participate in these programs by establishing a minimum standard of ethical care and operation. Individuals who adhere to these guidelines will be considered as upholding, contributing to, and promoting a high standard of operation and service.

1 Competence

Professionals strive to maintain high standards of competence in their work. They recognize the boundaries of their competencies and understand the potential limitations of adventure activities. Professionals exercise reasonable judgment and take appropriate precautions to promote the welfare of participants. They maintain knowledge of relevant professional information related to the use of adventure experiences and they recognize their need for ongoing education. Professionals make appropriate use of professional, technical, and administrative resources that serve the best interests of participants in their program.

1.1 Boundaries of competence

(a) Professionals provide services only within the boundaries of their competence, based on their education, training, supervision, experience, and practice. (b) Professionals provide services involving specific practices after first undertaking appropriate study, training, supervision, and/or consultation from persons who are competent in those areas or practices. (c) In those areas where generally recognized standards for preparatory training do not yet exist, professionals take reasonable steps to ensure the competence of their work and to promote the welfare of participants. (d) Professionals seek appropriate assistance for their personal problems or conflicts that may impair their work performance or judgment.

1.2 Continuing training

Professionals are aware of current information in their fields of activity and undertake ongoing professional efforts to maintain the knowledge, practice, and skills they use at a competent level.

2 Integrity

Professionals seek to promote integrity in the practice of adventure programming. In these experiences, they are honest, fair, and respect others. In describing or reporting their qualifications, services, products, fees, and research, professionals do not make statements that are false, misleading, or deceptive. Professionals strive to be aware of their own belief systems, values, needs, and limitations and the effect of these on their work.

2.1 Interaction with other professionals

In deciding whether to offer or provide services to those already receiving services elsewhere, professionals carefully consider the potential participant's welfare. Professionals discuss these issues with participants in order to minimize the risk of confusion and conflict, consult with other professionals when appropriate, and proceed with caution and sensitivity. Professionals do not engage, directly or through agents, in uninvited solicitation of services from actual or potential participants or others who, because of particular circumstances, are vulnerable to undue influences (e.g., respecting client relationships).

2.2 Supervision

Professionals delegate to their employees, supervisees, or students only those professional responsibilities that such persons can perform competently. Within the limitations of their individual or other roles, professionals provide proper training or supervision to employees or supervisees. Professionals also take reasonable steps to see that such persons perform these services responsibly, competently, and ethically.

3 Professional responsibility

Professionals uphold ethical principles of conduct, clarify their roles and obligations, accept responsibility for their behavior and decisions, and adapt their methods to the needs of different populations. Professionals consult with, refer to, and cooperate with other professionals and individuals to the full extent needed to serve the best interests of participants. Professionals are concerned about the ethical professional conduct of their colleagues. When appropriate, they consult with colleagues in order to avoid unethical conduct. Because of its direct negative influence on participants as well as the field, professionals are strongly urged to report alleged unethical behavior to appropriate and pre-scribed channels. Professionals are ethically bound to cooperate with profes-sional associations' inquiries concerning ethical misconduct.

3.1 Basis for professional judgments

Professionals have an adequate basis for their professional judgments and actions that are derived from professional knowledge.

3.2 Initiation and length of services

Professionals do not begin services for individuals where the constraints of limited contact will not benefit the participant. Professionals continue services only as long as it is reasonably clear that participants are benefit-ing from those services.

3.3 Concern for the environment

Professionals conduct adventure experiences in a manner that has minimal impact on the environment. Professionals do not conduct adventure experiences where permanent damage to wilderness environments will occur as a result of programming.

4 Respect for people's rights and dignity

Professionals respect the fundamental rights, dignity, and worth of all people. They respect the rights of individuals to privacy, confidentiality, and self-deter-mination. Professionals strive to be sensitive to cultural and individual differ-ences, including those due to age, gender, race, ethnicity, national origin, religion, sexual preference, disability, and socioeconomic status. Professionals do not engage in sexual or other harassment or exploitation of participants, students, trainees, supervisees, employees, colleagues, research subjects, or actual or potential witnesses or complainants in investigations and ethical proceedings.

4.1 Policy against discrimination

Professionals do not discriminate against or refuse professional services to anyone on the basis of age, gender, race, ethnicity, national origin, religion, sexual preference, disability, or socioeconomic status.

4.2 Ethic of empowerment

Professionals respect the rights of participants to make decisions and help them to understand the consequences of their choices. Professionals assist participants in charting the course of their own lives. They respect the rights of participants to make decisions affecting their lives that also demonstrate an equal concern for the rights of others.

4.3 Describing the nature and results of adventure programming

When professionals provide services to individuals or groups, they first provide the consumer of services with appropriate information about the nature of such services and their rights, risks, and responsibilities. Professionals also provide an opportunity to discuss the results, interpretations, and conclusions with participants.

4.4 Informed consent

Professionals respect participants' rights to refuse or consent to services and activities. Participants must be well informed of the fees, confidentiality, benefits, risks, and responsibilities associated with these services and activities prior to participation. Professionals make reasonable efforts to answer participants' questions, avoid apparent misunderstanding about the service, and avoid creating unrealistic expectations in participants. Professionals inform participants of the relevant limitations of confidentiality as early as possible and the foreseeable uses of the information generated through their services. In the case of participants who are minors, parents and/or legal guardians must also give informed consent for participation. Professionals obtain informed consent from participants, parents, or guardians before videotaping, audio recording, or permitting third-party observation.

4.5 Fees

Professionals charge appropriate fees for services. Fees are disclosed to participants at the beginning of services and are truthfully represented to participants and third-party payers. Professionals are not guided solely by a desire for monetary reimbursement. They are encouraged to contribute a portion of their professional time for little or no personal advantage.

4.6 Advertisement

Professionals accurately represent their competence, training, education, and experience relevant to their practices. This practice includes using: (1) Titles that inform participants and the public about the true and accurate identity, responsibility, source, and status of those practicing under that title. (2) Professional identification (e.g., business card, office sign, letter-head, or listing) that does not include statements that are false, fraudulent, deceptive, or misleading.

4.7 Distortion of information by others

Professionals make efforts to prevent the distortion or misuse of their clinical materials and research findings. Professionals correct, whenever possible, false, inaccurate, or misleading information and representations made by others concerning their qualifications, services, or products.

4.8 Public opinions and recommendations

Professionals, because of their ability to influence and alter the lives of others and the field, exercise special care when making public their professional recommendations and opinions (e.g., public statements and testimony).

5 Concern for welfare

Professionals are sensitive to real and ascribed differences in power between themselves and their participants, and they avoid exploiting or misleading other people during or after professional relationships.

5.1 Professional relationships

Professionals provide services only in the context of a defined professional relationship or role.

5.2 Dual relationships

Professionals are aware of their influential position with respect to parti-cipants and avoid exploiting the trust and dependency of such persons. Because of this, professionals make every effort to avoid dual relationships with participants that could impair professional judgment (e.g., business or close personal relationships with participants). When dual relationships exist, professionals take appropriate professional precautions to ensure that judgment is not impaired and no exploitation occurs.

5.3 Sexual relationships

Sexual intimacy with participants is prohibited during the time of the professional relationship. Professionals engaging in sexual intimacy with past participants bear the burden of proving that there is no form of exploitation occurring.

5.4 Physical contact

Adventure activities often include various forms of physical contact between professionals and participants or among participants (e.g., spotting, checking climbing harnesses, holding hands). Professionals are sensitive and respectful of the fact that participants experience varying degrees of comfort with physical contact, even when it is offered for safety, encouragement, or support. Whenever possible, professionals inform, explain, and gain consent for usual and customary forms of physical contact. Professionals are aware of individual needs when initiating physical contact, especially if the contact is meant to communicate support (e.g., hugs, pats) and is otherwise not required for a particular activity. Except when safety is a factor, participants have the right to limit or refuse physical contact with professionals and participants.

5.5 Behavior management

Each program and professional will approach the topic of managing behavior with a concern for dignity and safety for both participants and professionals. Definitions of appropriate and inappropriate behaviors of participants should be made clear to participants before any adventure programming commences. Professional responses to inappropriate behaviors should be clearly understood by both professionals and participants and carried out in an appropriate manner. There should be clear documentation of staff training and awareness about program policies concerning the management of unsafe behavior. Policies should never advocate the use of restraint unless participant(s) impose a threat to themselves or others. Restraint should never be used as a punishment or to frighten, humiliate, or threaten a participant. Whenever possible, restraint should be avoided and as passive as possible. All behavior management should be accurately documented.

5.6 Physical needs of participants

Participants will be provided with the necessary water, nutrition, clothing, shelter, or other essential needs for the environment they are living in, unless there is a prior mutual consent between participants and professionals and it is recognized that this will serve a valid purpose (e.g., solo). At no time during any program will the withholding of these needs be used as a punitive measure.

5.7 Physical treatment of participants

At no time will participants be asked to perform excessive physical activity as a means of punishment. There should be a direct relationship between the participants' physical activity levels and the objective of the experience.

5.8 Appropriate use of risk

The amount of actual emotional and physical risk participants experience in adventure activities will be appropriate for the objectives and competence level of participants. Professionals use appropriate judgment when choosing activities that expose participants to actual or perceived physical and emotional risks.

5.9 Assisting participants in obtaining alternative services

Professionals assist participants in obtaining other services if they are unwilling or unable, for appropriate reasons, to provide professional help. Professionals will not unilaterally terminate services to participants without making reasonable attempts to arrange for the continuation of such services (e.g., referral). Experiences are planned with the intent that decisions made during and after the experience are in accordance with the best interest of participants.

5.10 Confidentiality

Professionals respect the right of participants to decide the extent to which confidential material is made public. Professionals may not disclose participant confidences except: (a) as mandated by law; (b) to prevent a clear and immediate danger to a person or persons; (c) where the professional is a defendant in civil, criminal, or disciplinary action arising from services (in which case participant confidences may be disclosed only in the course of that action); or (d) if there is a waiver previously obtained in writing, and then such information may be revealed only in accordance with the terms of the waiver. Unless it is contraindicated or not feasible, the discussion of confidentiality occurs at the onset of the professional relationship.

5.11 Use of case materials with teaching or professional presentations

Professionals only use participant or clinical materials in teaching, writing, and public presentations if a written waiver has been obtained in accordance with guideline 5.10 or when appropriate steps have been taken to disguise participant identity and assure confidentiality.

5.12 Storage and disposal of participant materials

Professionals store and dispose of participant records in ways that maintain confidentiality. Records should be maintained for a minimum of seven (7) years, or as mandated by state licensing boards, whichever is longer.

6 Social responsibility

Professionals are aware of their professional responsibilities to the community and society in which they work and live. Within the limitations of their roles, professionals avoid the misuse of their work. Professionals comply with the standards and laws in their particular geographical and professional area. Professionals also encourage the development of standards and policies that serve the interests of participants and the public.

*Adapted from the original work of the Therapeutic Adventure Professional Group Ethics Committee, 1991, https://www.aee.org/ethical-guidelines-for-ccat.

References

Alcoholics Anonymous World Services. (1957). *Alcoholics Anonymous comes of age: A brief history of A. A.* New York: Alcoholics Anonymous World Services, Inc.

Alvarez, T.*et al.* (2021). *Adventure group psychotherapy: An experiential approach to treatment.* New York: Routledge.

American Psychiatric Association. (2022). *Diagnostic and statistical manual of mental disorders* (5th edn., text rev.). Washington, DC: American Psychiatric Publishing, Inc.

Aubry, P. (2009). *Stepping stones: A therapeutic adventure activity guide.* Beverly, MA: Project Adventure.

Bacon, S. (1983). *The conscious use of metaphor in Outward Bound.* Denver, CO: Colorado Outward Bound School.

Bacon, S. (1987). *The evolution of the Outward Bound process.* Greenwich, CT: Outward Bound, Inc. (ERIC Reproduction Service No. Ed 295 780).

Bacon, S. and Kimball, R. (1989). The wilderness challenge model. In R. D. Lyman (Ed.), *Residential and inpatient treatment of children and adolescents.* NY: Plenum Press.

Bacon, S. B. (1991). Using the ropes course to help alcoholics resist temptation. In M. A. Gass and C. H. Dobkin (Eds.), *Book of metaphors: Volume I.* Available from editors at University of New Hampshire, Durham, NH, 11–12.

Bateson, G. (2002). *Mind and nature: A necessary unity.* New York: Hampton.

Bell, B. J., & Williams, B. G. (2006). Learning from first-year fears: An analysis of the Harvard first-year outdoor program's "fear in a hat" exercise. *Journal of college orientation, transition, and retention,* 14(1). doi:10.24926/jcotr.v14i1.2654.

Black, D. (2008). An effective strategy for improving physical & mental health. *Mindfulness: Clinical science insights,* 7.

Bostick, K., & Lottig, B. (2022). *Kitori.* https://www.kikoriapp.com.

Bouchrika, I. (2023, October 31). *50 Current student stress statistics: 2023 data analysis & predictions.* Research.com. https://rb.gy/9x7ddt.

Boyton, T. (1970). *Reach, touch and teach: Student concerns and process education.* New York: McGraw-Hill.

Brown, M. (2010). Transfer: outdoor adventure education's Achilles heel? Changing participation as a viable option, *Australian Journal of Outdoor Education,* 14(1), 13+.

CDC. (2023, March). Centers for Disease Control and Prevention. *Data and statistics on children's mental health*. Children's Mental Health. https://www.cdc.gov/childrensmentalhealth/data.html.

Cecchin, G. (1987). Hypothesizing, circularity, and neutrality revisited: an invitation to curiosity. *Family processes*, 26(4), 405–413.

Chalquist, C. (2009). A look at the ecopsychology research evidence, *Ecopsychology*, 1(2), 1–11.

Child Focus. (2022, April 4). *Mental health in childhood: Undiagnosed and silently suffering*. https://rb.gy/427srw.

Curtin, S. C. (2020). State suicide rates among adolescents and young adults aged 10–24: United States, 2000–2018. *Centers for Disease Control and Prevention: National vital statistics reports*, 11(69), 1–10.

de Shazer, S. (1982). *Patterns of brief family therapy*. New York: Guilford Press.

Dewey, J. (1938). *Experience and education*. New York: Free Press.

Doherty, K. (1995). A qualitative analysis of three teaching styles. *Journal of experiential education*, 18(1), 18–22.

Donnellan, H., & Jack, G. (2014). Four stages of the experiential learning cycle, *The survival guide for newly qualified social workers* (2nd edn.). Philadelphia, PA: Jessica Kingsley Publishers.

Durgin, C. H., & McEwen, D. (1991). Troubled young people after the adventure program. *Journal of experiential education*, 14(1), 31–35.

Eisenberg, D., & Neighbors, K. (2007). *Economic and policy issues in preventing mental disorders and substance abuse among young people: Presentation for the IOM Committee on the Prevention of Mental Disorders and Substance Abuse*, October 31st, 2007: Department of Health Management and Policy School of Public Health. University of Michigan.

Ewert, A. (1990). Research update: Revisiting the concept of self-esteem through outdoor experiential activities. *Journal of Experiential Education*, 13(2), 56.

Frank, L. (2001). *Journey toward the caring classroom: Using adventure to create community* (2nd edn.). Bethany, OK: Woods "N" Barnes.

Frankl, V. E. (1946). *Man's search for meaning*. Boston, MA: Beacon Press.

Freedman, J., & Combs, G. *Narrative therapy: The social construction of preferred realities*. New York and London: W.W. Norton and Company.

Gass, M. A. (1986). Programming the transfer of learning in adventure education. *Journal of experiential education*, 8(3), 18–24.

Gass, M. A. (1990). The longitudinal effects of an adventure orientation program. *Journal of experiential education*, 31(1), 33–38.

Gass, M. A. (1991). Enhancing metaphoric transfer in adventure therapy programs. *Journal of experiential education*, 14(2), 6–13.

Gass, M. (1993). *Therapeutic applications of adventure programming*. Dubuque, IA: Kendall Hunt Publishing Company.

Gass, M. (1995). *Book of Metaphors: A descriptive presentation of metaphors for adventure activities – Volume 2*. Dubuque, IA: Kendall Hunt Publishing Company.

Gass, M. A. (1997). Facilitating experiential learning: Co-creating stories with better endings for clients. *Journal of Experiential Education*, 20(2), 66–67.

Gass, M. A., & Dobkin, C. H. (Eds.) (1991). *Book of Metaphors: Volume I*. Dubuque, IA: Kendall Hunt Publishing Company.

Gass, M.A., Garvey, D., & Sugerman, D. (2003). The long-term effects of a first-year student wilderness orientation program. *Journal of experiential education*, 26(1), 34–40.

Gass, M.A., & Gillis, H. L. (1995). CHANGES: A model using adventure experiences as assessment. *Journal of experiential education*, 18(1), 34–40.

Gass, M.A., & Gillis, H. L. (2010). ENHANCES: Adventure therapy supervision. *Journal of experiential education*, 33(1), 72–89.

Gass, M. A., Gillis, H. L., & Russell, K. (2020). *Adventure therapy. Theory, practice, & research*. Second Edition. New York: Routledge.

Gass, M.A., & Priest, S. (1993). Using metaphors and isomorphs to enhance the transfer of learning in adventure education. *Journal of adventure education*, 10(4), 18–24.

Gass, M. A., & Priest, S. (2006). Effectiveness of metaphoric facilitation styles in corporate adventure training (CAT) programs. *Journal of experiential education, 29(1)*, 18–24.

Gillis, H. L. (1986). *An exploratory study comparing the strategic use of metaphorical introductions with traditional introductions in a one-day adventure workshop for couples' enrichment* (unpublished doctoral dissertation). The University of Georgia. Dissertation Abstracts International, 47/09- A, 3312.

Gillis, H. L., & Bonney, W. C. (1986). Group counselling with couples or families: Adding adventure activities. *Journal for specialists in group work*, 11(4), 213–219.

Gillis, H. L., & Gass, M. A. (2010). Residential treatment of juveniles in a sex offender program using an adventure-based behavioral management program: A matched group design. *Journal of Child Sex Abuse*, 19(1), 20–34.

Gillis, H. L., Gass, M. A., & Russell, K. (2008). The effectiveness of Project Adventure's behavior management programs for male offenders in residential treatment. *Residential treatment for children and youth*, 25(3), 227–247.

Gillis, H. L., & Hirsch, J. (1998). *Developing metaphors for group activities*. Milledgeville. GA: Georgia College.

Hager, P. (2008). Learning and metaphors. *Medical teacher*, 30(7), 679–686.

Haley, J. (1973). *Uncommon therapy: The psychiatric techniques of M. Milton Erikson, M.D.* New York: W. W. Norton & Company.

Haley, J. (1988). *Problem-solving therapy*. San Francisco, CA: Jossey-Bass Publishers.

Hirsch, J., & Gillis, H. L. (2004). *Developing metaphors for group activities*. [DVD]. Boulder, CO: Association for Experiential Education.

Hofstadter, D. (1979). *Gödel, Escher, Bach: An eternal golden braid*. New York: Basic Books.

Hunter, M. (1986). *Teach for transfer*. El Segundo, CA: TIP Publications.

Itin, C. (1995). Utilizing hypnotic language in adventure therapy. *Journal of experiential education*, 18(2), 70–75.

Itin, C. M. (2001). Adventure therapy—critical questions. *Journal of experiential education*, 24(2), 80–84.

Kabbat-Zinn, J. (2003). Mindfulness-based interventions in context: Past, present, and future. *Clinical psychology: Science and practice*, 10(2), 144–156.

Kaplan, R., & Kaplan, S. (1993). *Experience of nature*. New York: Cambridge University Press.

Kimball, R. O. (1983). The wilderness as therapy. *Journal of experiential education*, 6(3), 6–9.

Kirkpatrick, D. L. (1994). *Evaluating training programs – The four levels.* San Francisco, CA: Berrett-Koehler Publishers, Inc.

Kjol, R., & Weber, J. (1990). The 4th fire: Adventure-based counseling with juvenile sex offenders. *Journal of experiential education*, 13(3), 18–22.

Kolb, D. (1984). *Experiential learning: Experience as the source of learning and development.* Englewood Cliffs, NJ: Prentice-Hall.

Lung, D. M., *et al.* (2008). *Power of one: Using adventure and experiential activities within one-on-one counseling sessions.* Oklahoma City, OK: Wood "N" Barnes Publishing.

Mack, H. (1996). Inside work, outdoors: Women, metaphor, and meaning. In K. Warren (Ed.), *Women's voices in experiential education.* Boulder, CO: Association for Experimental Education.

MacRea, S., Moore, C., Savage, G., Soehner, D., & Priest, S. (1993). Changes in risk-taking propensity due to ropes course challenges. *Journal of adventure education and outdoor leadership*, 10(2), 10–12.

Mason, B. (2010). Psychodrama: Family sculpting. *Good therapy.* https://www.goodtherapy.org/blog/psychodrama-family-sculpting/.

Minuchin, S. (1981). *Family therapy techniques.* Cambridge, MA: Harvard University Press.

Moos, R. H., & Humphrey, B. (1974). *Group Environment Scale.* Palo Alto, CA: CPP.

Nadler, R. S., & Luckner, J. L. (1997). *Processing the adventure experience.* Dubuque, Iowa: Kendall-Hunt.

National Association of Social Workers of Maine. (2020). *Kinesthetic metaphor.* https://www.youtube.com/watch?v=XmXcZO6jpcA.

NATSAP. (2022). National Association for Therapeutic Schools and Programs. *The nuts & bolts of the golden thread.* The Golden Thread. https://www.youtube.com/watch?v=9f1SIwnhybY.

NSDUH. (2019, September). National Survey of Drug Use and Health. *Key Substance Use and Mental Health Indicators in the United States: Results from the 2019 National Survey on Drug Use and Health.* Substance Abuse and Mental Health Services Administration (SAMHSA). https://shorturl.at/lty35.

Otani, A. (1989). The Confusion Technique untangled: Its theoretical rationale and preliminary classification. *American journal of clinical hypnosis*, 31(3), 164–172.

Porter, W. (1989). *The development and evaluation of a therapeutic wilderness program for youth* (unpublished master's thesis). University of Denver, Denver, CO.

Priest, S., & Gass, M. (2005). *Effective leadership in adventure programming* (2nd edn.). Champaign: IL, Human Kinetics Publishing.

Priest, S., & Gass, M. A. (2018). *Effective leadership in adventure programming* (3rd edn.). Champaign, IL: Human Kinetics Publishing.

Priest, S., & Gass, M., Gillis, H. L. (2009). *Essential elements of facilitation: Skills for enhancing client.* Vancouver, BC: TARRAK Publications.

Prochaska, J. O., & Velicer, W. F. (1997) The transtheoretical model of health behavior change. *American journal of health promotion*, 12(1), 38–48.

Prochaska, J. O., & Norcross, J. C. (2002). Stages of change. In J. Norcross (Ed.), *Psychotherapy relationships that work: Therapist contributions and responsiveness to patients.* NY: Oxford University Press.

Rohnke, K. (1984). *Silver bullets.* Hamilton, MA: Project Adventure, Inc.

Rohnke, K. (1988). Personal communication with author.

Rohnke, K. (1989). *Cowstails and cobras* II (103–104). Hamilton, MA: Project Adventure, Inc.

Rohnke, K., & Butler, S. (1995). *Quicksilver*. Beverly, MA: Project Adventure.

Rossi, E. L. (Ed.). (1980). *The collected papers of Milton H. Erickson on hypnosis*. New York: Penguin.

Rossi, E. L. (Ed.). (2008–2010). *The collective works of Milton H. Erickson*. New York: MHE Press.

Roszak, T. (2001). *The voice of the earth: An exploration of ecopsychology*. Grand Rapids, MI: Phanes Press.

Russell, K., & Farnum, J. (2004). A concurrent model of wilderness therapy process. *Journal of adventure education and outdoor learning*, 4(1), 39–55.

Russell, K. C., Gillis, H. L., & Heppner, W. (2015). An examination of mindfulness-based experiences through adventure in substance use disorder treatment for young adult males: A pilot study. *Mindfulness*, 7, 320–328.

Russell, K., & Gillis, H. L. (2017). The Adventure Therapy Experience Scale: The psychometric properties of a scale to measure the unique factors moderating an adventure therapy experience. *Journal of experiential education*, 40(2), 135–152. doi:10.1177/1053825917690541.

Satir, V. (1972/1990 (reissue)). *Peoplemaking*. Guildford, Surrey: Souvenir Press Ltd.

Schoel, J., & Maizell, R. (2002). *Islands of healing*. Hamilton, MA: Project Adventure, Inc.

Schoel, J., Prouty, D., & Radcliff, P. (1988). *Islands of healing: A guide to adventure-based counseling*. Hamilton, MA: Project Adventure, Inc.

Selye, H. (1974). *Stress without distress*. New York: Signet Books.

SAMHSA. (2020). Substance Abuse and Mental Health Services Administration. *Key substance use and mental health indicators in the United States: Results from the 2019 National survey on drug use and health* (HHS Publication No. PEP20–07–01–001, NSDUH Series H-55). Rockville, MD: Center for Behavioral Health Statistics and Quality, Substance Abuse and Mental Health Services Administration. https://www.samhsa.gov/data/.

Sutton, J. (2021, April 21). Client resistance in therapy: How to help difficult clients. *Positive Psychology*. https://positivepsychology.com/resistance-to-change/.

Tobler, N. S. (1986). Meta-analysis of 143 drug prevention programs. Quantitative outcome results of program participants compared to a control or comparison group. *Journal of drug issues*. 16(4), 537–567.

UNICEF. (2022, October 10). *On world mental health day, a plea for investing in more and better data*. UNICEF for every child. https://rb.gy/h61d28.

Unsoeld, W. (1976). *The spiritual values of the wilderness*. Miami, FL: Association for Experiential Education.

Walsh, V., & Golins, G. (1976). *Exploration of the Outward Bound process*. Denver, CO: Colorado Outward Bound School.

Walter, J. L., & Peller, J. E. (1992). *Becoming solution focused in brief therapy*. New York: Brunner/Mazel, Inc.

Waltzlawick, P., Weakland, J., & Fisch, R. (1978). *Change: Principles of problem formation and problem resolution*. New York: Norton.

Webster, S. (1988). *Safety standards for ropes course element and initiatives*. Hamilton, MA: Project Adventure.

Whitaker, C. (1978). *The family crucible: The intense experience of family therapy*. New York: Harper and Row.

White, M., & Epston, D. (1990). *Narrative means to therapeutic ends*. New York: W.W. Norton.

Zeig, J. (Ed.). (1992). *The evolution of psychotherapy: The second conference*. New York: Routledge.

Zeig, J. (Ed.). (1994). *Ericksonian methods: The essence of the story*. New York: Brunner-Mazel.

Zull, J. E. (2011). *From brain to mind: Using neuroscience to guide change in education*. New York: Taylor & Francis Group.

Index